Plan For Rapid Weight Loss

This book includes

The Autophagy Diet

Intermittent Fasting For Women

Table of Contents

Chapter 7: Different Goals and Reasons for Using Autophagy and Low Carb Eating in Life   174

Chapter 8: Frequently Asked Questions, Tips, and Encouragement for Long-Term Success and Benefits of the Autophagy Diet   177

Intermittent Fasting for Women

A Beginner's Guide for Rapid Weight Loss, Burning Fat, Improving Overall Health and Minimizing the Effect of Aging in a Scientific Way

Introduction

Congratulations on downloading *Intermittent Fasting for Women* and thank you for doing so! I'm sure you've heard a lot about intermittent fasting and its role in fixing health problems and maintaining wholeness. One of the reasons intermittent fasting continues to spread like wildfire among both women and men is the fact it helps to shed off excess weight.

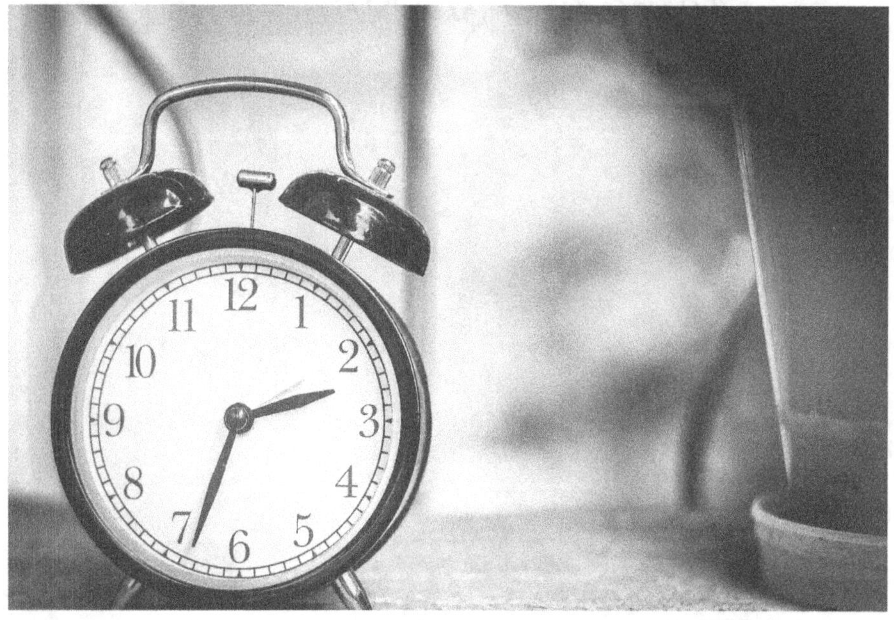

Let's face it; losing weight and fat is tough. By the time you're downloading this book, you probably have tried all manner of diets that have yielded little or no results. Even worse, most of these diets are expensive; hence, they are out of reach for an average working person. Rather, intermittent fasting is more promising. Intermittent fasting involves making a lifestyle change, especially with your feeding pattern, where you cycle between periods of eating and fasting. Intermittent fasting will not cost you more than you'd normally spend on meals. In fact, it could be less. This diet is designed to enhance the burning of excess fat and helping you lead a healthy lifestyle. When done properly, you will achieve success with intermittent fasting.

In this book, I introduce to you the intermittent fasting way of life and explain how you can tap into it as a woman to reap maximum results. Most books written about intermittent fasting ignore the fact that the female body is unique hence responds to intermittent fasting differently. They also don't take into account the impact of fasting on a woman's hormonal balance. This book focuses on how you benefit from intermittent fasting as a woman and embrace it without running into health problems!

Chapter 1: What is Intermittent Fasting?

Intermittent fasting refers to a pattern of eating where you alternate between defined periods of eating and fasting. Intermittent fasting emphasizes on when you eat as opposed to what you eat. As such, there are various intermittent fasting methods that you can adapt depending on your lifestyle and other factors. From staying for extended periods without food to skipping a meal, there are various variations of intermittent fasting. However, you may consume non-caloric beverages, including tea, coffee, and water. Intermittent fasting offers a number of benefits that have seen an increase in the number of people embracing this as a lifestyle.

History of Fasting

Intermittent fasting is not a new concept. It's an ancient tradition that is time tested. The history of dating goes back to more than a thousand years ago. Human beings have fasted either out of necessity due to food scarcity or for religious reasons. The only new thing about it is the extensive research that has been done highlighting the effects of intermittent fasting. Fasting cuts across varied and multiple traditions for health or spiritual reasons. Although out of necessity, fasting was a common practice among the hunters and gatherers who didn't have cold storage and modern food preservation methods. Thus, they were forced to go for extended periods without food until they found something.

Greek philosopher Hippocrates, the father of medicine advocated for fasting. He held the belief that eating when you're sick is akin to feeding your illness. Plato and Plutarch were equally advocates of fasting. Greeks held the belief that since sick animals didn't eat the same should apply to humans. They were convinced that fasting didn't just improve the cognitive function but also healed illnesses. This has been advanced into modern medicine, especially prior to surgery. Fasting is also a spiritual practice among various religions as it is believed to provide mental, physical, and spiritual benefits. Some of the religious fasting practices like Ramadhan among the Muslims observe intermittent fasting patterns.

Today, intermittent fasting continues to gain attention, especially among people who are conscious about their health and general wellbeing. This practice was popularized by Dr. Michael Mosley, a BBC journalist who fasted for two days every week in 2012 and posted tremendous results among them rapid weight loss. He highlighted these benefits on his program the popularity of the trend. Dr. Mosley has also written a book on intermittent fasting. Today, there are numerous ways of doing intermittent fasting that produce amazing benefits. Intermittent fasting is a fairly easy practice to follow that will leave you feeling better and more energetic. You'll be surprised that hunger will no longer be an issue because your body gets used to going for defined periods without food.

Who's Intermittent Fasting For?

Intermittent fasting is not a preserve of fitness enthusiasts. If anything we all practice some form of fasting, albeit unknowingly. The only difference is that when you're deliberate about intermittent fasting, you have clearly defined the duration of your fast and feast intervals. According to data from clinical research, intermittent fasting can contribute to extending lifespan, regulating blood glucose, reducing the risk of coronary disease, controlling blood lipids, managing bodyweight and reducing the risk of cancers among other benefits.

Thus, intermittent fasting can be practiced by just about everyone except individuals with special needs. This means that it's not something that you'll do randomly and expect to reap all the benefits listed above. Intermittent fasting requires you to be disciplined in adhering to the eating pattern of your choice. Even then, you must pay attention to your nutritional specifics. You're most likely have success with intermittent fasting if; you're single or don't have children, have a history of monitoring your food/calorie intake, or you have a job that allows periods of low performance. These conditions make it easy to transition into intermittent fasting and make it a lifestyle.

Who Should Avoid Intermittent Fasting?

Intermittent fasting is not for everyone. For some people, incorporating the pattern of eating that includes periods of fasting might be troublesome or inconvenient. Some pre-existing conditions can make it harder to do intermittent fasting. If the risks of practicing intermittent fasting outweigh the potential benefits, then it is not for you, and you'll have to refrain from practicing it. Some of the people who should avoid intermittent fasting include:

Expectant and breastfeeding mothers. You shouldn't even think of intermittent fasting if you're pregnant or are breastfeeding. It's obvious that during this time, both you and your baby need to be well-nourished and healthy. Moreover, you also need more calories during pregnancy and when you're breastfeeding.

Young people under 18 years old. At this age, you're still growing; hence, you require all the vital nutrients and minerals for your growth and development as such, you need to refrain from practicing intermittent fasting.

People who are malnourished and underweight. It's almost impossible to imagine that a person who is underweight or you have an eating disorder will want to take part in intermittent fasting. If you're not sure whether you're malnourished or not consider talking to a physician or even calculate your BMI. It's also advisable that you stay away from intermittent fasting if you're struggling with an eating disorder because it could just worsen it.

People with gastroesophageal reflux disease (GERD). A number of studies have shown that GERD can be aggravated by fasting. This is attributed to the fact that during fasting, your stomach stays without food, so there's nothing left for gastric juices to digest.

Other categories of people who should avoid intermittent fasting include those who are chronically stressed have previously suffered from disordered eating, you are getting into a diet and exercise regimen, or you simply don't sleep well.

Who Should Approach Intermittent Fasting With Caution?

Some of the people who approach intermittent fasting with caution include the following:

You're taking medication. When you're taking medication, you must be careful so that it doesn't overlap with your fasting period. This is particularly important for medications that require that you eat before taking your medication.

Individuals with Type 2 diabetes. If you're suffering from type 2 diabetes, it's advisable that you talk to your physician before attempting intermittent fasting.

Patients on cancer therapy. Cancer therapy and other related medical treatment can be brutal to your body. As such, you must approach intermittent fasting with caution. In fact, make sure that you speak to your physician before you begin intermittent fasting.

What Happens When You Fast?

When your body is operating normally, it relies on the glucose that is stored in the muscles and liver for energy. However, when these stores are exhausted, it goes into a state known as ketosis. That is, the liver will break down fat, producing ketones that can then be used as a source of energy. There's evidence to the effect that ketones have the ability to trigger a reduction of appetite as well as reduce inflammation levels and oxidative stress. Even then, ketones are not only a source of energy, but they also offer numerous other benefits. Therefore, when you fast, you reduce the risk factors for certain conditions like heart disease and type 2 diabetes.

Conversely, there are certain disadvantages associated with eating and digestion, especially if your food contains free radicals. Well, this is not to say that it's wrong to eat; rather, taking a rest from eating will give your body rest from these processes. A number of studies done, taking into consideration diabetes risk factors like appetite hormones, blood glucose levels, and other relevant markers showed improvements associated with time-restricted eating.

What Makes Intermittent the Best Way to Lose Fat?

If you're like other women who are struggling to lose excessive fat and maintain a lean body, then you definitely want to try out intermittent fasting. But just what is it that makes intermittent the best way to lose weight? To being with, you need to understand that intermittent fasting isn't a product, rather it's more of adopting a lifestyle change around your eating habits. Thus, it's more of a natural process that results in weight loss as well as a loss of visceral fat.

Simply put, intermittent fasting lets your body burn fat naturally but only when you're determined and disciplined because you'll have to learn to make conscious decisions about your lifestyle and eating choices. Since there are no changes that involve steroid or chemical changes, the results take time depending on the intermittent fasting protocol you'll adopt.

Intermittent fasting continues to deliver results for many people several years after gaining popularity because of its simple to follow through yet has the ability to deliver results. You don't need to do anything special to incorporate it into your lifestyle. All you have to do is fast and do it intermittently. That is, create a gap in your fasting and eating schedule to bring about a significant change. Thus, there's a lot of excitement around this pattern of eating because while diets have dominated the wellness industry for years, the results of intermittent fasting are tremendous. Besides, most diets tend to be restrictive; hence, you will often look forward to the end of the diet period to go back to your regular eating plan. Diets tend to create a temptation that is often seen as a counterforce as you're constantly thinking about the foods you can't eat. As such, it's not uncommon for most people to get into binge eating soon after getting off a diet. In fact, evidence points to the fact that over 80% of people who followed a diet with the goal of losing weight ended up gaining the weight they lost or even more.

On the contrary, intermittent fasting is more relaxed and easy to embrace because it only imposes restrictions on the time when you get to eat. That is, it puts a limitation and an emphasis on the hours of eating as opposed to the kinds of foods you can eat. This eliminates the possibility of having cravings or even binge eating. This makes it possible for you to burn more fat hence become leaner and healthier. It's a holistic approach to staying healthy and fit.

Why You Should Start Intermittent Fasting?

There's nothing unusual about going without food for a stipulated period. If anything, the human body is well wired to handle extended periods of fasting. Your body is capable of surviving for up to 84 hours before you begin experiencing a significant drop in your glucose. There's so much that goes on in your body when you fast. The good news is that most of these changes have a positive impact on your overall wellbeing. Fasting creates a conducive environment for certain repair processes that include hormones, genes, and cells.

Moreover, when your body is in the fasted state, you'll experience a significant decrease in insulin and blood sugar levels as well as an increase in the human growth hormone. Intermittent fasting is also a great way to increase your metabolic health benefits by improving a number of health markers and risk factors. Intermittent fasting is also believed to contribute towards increasing longevity by extending your lifespan.

Intermittent fasting also simplifies your day because you'll require less time and probably spend less money on your meals. While you'd ordinarily have to prepare up to six meals in a day, this can be reduced to just two. You'll be surprised how your body will get used to these changes over time. This is the concept that the hunter and gatherer communities lived by when there was scarcity. Overall, it's a life hack that will make your life simpler as well as improve your health.

Chapter 2: How Intermittent Fasting Works

Although most of the popular exercise and diet trends have their footing in legitimate science, the facts are usually distorted by the time they become popular. Instead, the benefits are distorted and overemphasized, while the risks are overlooked. Generally, science is made to take the back seat. This is same with intermittent fasting that has seen so many people jump in without really understanding the science behind it. In fact, intermittent fasting has become so popular that it might quickly become a fad.

Although mostly done on animals, research has been done backing the health benefits of incorporating fasting in your lifestyle. The results are quite promising as they are proof of the benefits of fasting such as improving biomarkers of disease, preserving memory and learning functioning, improving biomarkers of disease, and reduction of oxidative stress.

There are numerous theories about why intermittent fasting offers physiological benefits. The most studied is the hypothesis that when you're fasting, cells undergo minor stress that they respond to adaptively by improving their ability to cope with stress or even fight disease. Although stress often has a negative connotation, it doesn't always have to be negative. For instance, when you engage in vigorous exercise, your cardiovascular system and muscles are stressed. However, these become even stronger when given time to recover. There's a significant similarity between how cells respond to stress and intermittent fasting. Understanding the science behind intermittent fasting is the gateway to the smooth integration of this pattern of eating into your lifestyle and see the results.

The Basics of Fuel Burning

The human digestive system works in a balletic manner by communicating within itself constantly while checking on the physical state. As such, there's precision when it comes to the amount of food that is burned and converted into calories versus what is stored as fat. These processes are not random; thus if you want to lose fat, it is important that you begin by understanding how the system works. The body is used to being in intervals of the fed and fasted state. That is a time when the body has fuel (food) to burn and a time when you don't eat anything. When your body detects a drop in the level of food and energy, it begins to secrete ghrelin, the hunger hormone that signals the brain food is required. When you ignore this signal for an extended period, it translates into a hunger that you'll eventually be unable to ignore. Most of the hormonal production is linked to your eating production. For instance, if you eat at noon, your stomach will adjust to this schedule and remind you when it's time to eat.

Once this pattern is established, a certain effect develops so that should you eat earlier than noon, the food is burned and stored with the assumption that you'll refuel at noon. This means that when you change your meal times, your body will adjust the ration of burn versus store in compliance with the new environment. The aim of this process is to ensure a smooth transition from the fed and fasted states. In an ideal world, when you only eat when you're hungry, your body will maintain the status quo.

Insulin regulates and measures the transition between the fasted and fed state. Insulin is the body's way of knowing if you need to eat or not. Simply put, insulin is crucial in helping the body to survive through tough times. There's a specific order through which your body burns food in order to serve the immediate needs first and store the rest for a rainy day.

Priority is given to fuel generation is given to carbohydrates first. Carbohydrates can be drawn from vegetables and grains even though vegetables have smaller amounts. When you consume carbohydrates, they're converted to glucose which the body burns to give you energy. Glucose is good because it gives you instant energy. The second priority for fuel burning is given to fat. This is because the process of burning fat takes time and requires the body to use more energy. Therefore, when you ingest fat, it doesn't release energy instantaneously. Rather, it's delayed. Even then, fat is extremely important because it serves as a backup source of fuel. Thus, when you experience a shortage or even famine, your body begins by burning traces of glucose in the body, followed by body fat. It's only after exhausting these that it will then turn to muscles for energy.

Generally, the body would rather not burn muscles, which are major proteins, since this is what it is made of. As such, by burning muscles for fuel, it means your body is cannibalizing. Besides, muscles aren't great at energy delivery as a lot more has to be burned to generate the amount of energy you'd generate from fat/glucose. This is why muscle is not a preferred source of fuel.

To Store or to Burn?

Whenever you eat, your body makes a choice between how much food it will burn and how much it will store. This decision is influenced by your strength level, among other factors. The body's way of reasoning is such that the more the muscle, the stronger you're hence can withstand calamity better. Consequently, there's less need to store up fat for the rainy day. On the contrary, if you're weaker, you need to store fat within you to sustain you. This explains why you cannot lose fat/weight from starving alone. When you starve, the body enters a panic mode and burns the fat within your body. Additionally, it also burns muscles after a while so that you begin losing strength and become weak. However, when you begin eating post starvation, the body will first recognize the lack of strength and store more fat within you to account for this.

This also happens when you eat normally such that any excess carbs after your energy and glucose needs are met is converted into fat regardless of your levels of strength. This is the reason eating sugar makes you fat; once the energy needs are met, excess sugar is converted into fat for storage. Protein is diverted to muscles directly. When you consume carbs and fat, the carbs are burned to generate fuel while the fat is stored. Excess carbs are also stored. This essentially means that it's not fat that makes you fat but excessive carbs. These include sugars among other foods. This explains why the ketogenic diet works in promoting weight loss despite advocating for the consumption of high amounts of fat. However, this doesn't mean that you eat as much as you want rather, adhere to the basic principles.

Balancing Out

You may be asking yourself how you get to your body to burn more fat. It's simple. Your body will begin burning fat when it requires more fuel than what you're giving it. That is if the total amount of energy your drawing from carbs, protein, and fat is less than what your body requires, then it'll turn inward for fuel. When it burns glycogen/glucose, it becomes fat. This process is triggered when you have a caloric deficiency. This deficiency will cause your insulin levels to drop, making your body to burn stored fat because it's insulin that signals the body, whether it needs to wait for external fuel or seek within. A caloric deficit stimulates a fasted state. Consequently, if you need caloric surplus in order to put on weight because you'll be giving the body more than it actually needs. It's this phenomenon that intermittent fasting capitalizes on by increasing the amount of time your levels of insulin are low.

The Insulin Factor

In order to understand the science of intermittent fasting and what sets it apart from other weight loss plans, it's important that you first understand insulin and its role. As you may already know, insulin is a switch that determines the signals your body needs to either burn or store fat. What this means is that by keeping your insulin levels lower for longer, then you will burn more fat. Insulin levels will usually be low when you don't have an external source of fuel.

Conversely, insulin levels are high when you eat food. This means that your body doesn't burn internal fat when you eat. Keep in mind that starvation doesn't work when it comes to weight loss. Therefore, you need to work on striking a balance between starvation and managing your insulin levels so that they are at the right state. It's this balance that intermittent fasting establishes. That is, while your insulin spikes when you have a small eating window this food is mostly burned as fuel. The portion of food that is stored as fat is later burned during the long fasting period when your insulin level is low. Internal fat is also burned.

Intermittent fasting will not only help in lowering the level of insulin but also restore balance within you in relation to insulin resistance. People who can't stand being in a fasted state will grab something to eat whenever they feel slight hunger. Interestingly, the more you eat small meals throughout the day, the more you're bound to feel hungry. This shortens the fasting window. As a result, your body gets used to the idea of using up glycogen, thus hindering the burning of internal fat stores. When this happens, your body secrets more insulin keep burning the external glucose.

Consequently, your levels of insulin spike while your body fat continually increases, resulting in obesity. This is why obese people find it difficult to lose fat. Their bodies no longer remember how to burn fat. Instead, any changes they attempt to cause the body to fight back harder since it has forgotten how to burn fuel to get fuel. Thus, it's not surprising that a person who is overweight is likely to be hungrier than someone with a BMI that is within the normal range. A hunger that is driven by glucose is different in that it manifests through carb cravings that are difficult to resist. Overweight bodies change at a cellular level as the cells' smallest component that also burns fat adapts to burning glucose instead of the fat that is stored within the cell. Thus, an obese person will oscillate between being in a state of hunger and satiety.

Restoring the Balance

Being caught up in the cycle of being in a state of hunger and satiating often comes with other medical issues. When you realize this, you need to work towards breaking the cycle so that your body can go back to burning fat for fuel again. Although this transition is tougher if you're more dependent on glucose, none of the techniques of transitioning will be easy. There are a number of methods you can use in restoring insulin sensitivity and getting your body to be conscious to burning fat again. You can begin with a low carbohydrate diet. That is, you restrict the number of carbs you ingest so that your body has to burn fat because there is no other option. A ketogenic diet is a form of high-fat low carb diet.

You must beware of mental blocks that people have against high-fat diets because most of these are myths and poor advertising. By now, you know that fat has no role in putting on weight; rather; the problem lies with consuming excess carbs. High-intensity exercise is another great way of burning fat and glycogen. High-intensity exercise gets your heart pumping at a high rate so that your body is forced to burn the stored glycogen. Your body can begin to burn fat for fuel in order to continue. You can also consider adopting the caloric method where you eat less than you actually need so that you enforce a fast. Intermittent fasting is the last technique that is one of the easiest methods to implement because it allows your body an ample period of time to get used to burning fat. This is different from a keto diet that gives your body time to lower levels of insulin and burns fat but minimizes these chances by eating for most of the time in the day. Unlike keto, intermittent fasting that gives your body adequate time to restrict the time spent in the fed state. Spending more time in the fasted state gives your body time to burn glycogen and convert body fat into fuel. This means you don't have to pursue a low carb diet for intermittent fasting to work. However, combining the two is more effective. Alternating between fasting and the fed state sends your body into a form of metabolic exercise that forces your body to burn both fat and carbs. This trains the body to be good at both resulting in the better metabolization of food so that your body is not only reliant on a single type of food. The result of this is a decrease in the blood glucose and insulin levels while increasing insulin sensitivity, fatty acid mobilization, growth hormone production, and fat oxidation at the cellular level.

Although intermittent fasting is a great method by itself, it produces even better results when combined with decreased meal frequency and regular exercise. It's easy to assume that this method can only be effective when you spend more time fasting. The truth is that you need to find a balance so that you're not starved or overfed. Instead, cut on the number of times you're having in a day and include a workout routine that fits into your eating pattern. Exercising will get the heart pumping in addition to as well as aid fat loss. Your muscle mass helps to determine the division of the food you eat in terms of whether to burn as fuel or store. Thus, building muscle is the best way to lose fat. Women are hang-up against this because muscle building is often associated with bodybuilding, so they think their bodies will become like that. Thankfully, this view is debunked by the fact that women and men are biologically different. Hence, the way your body reacts to workout is different from how a man's body reacts. Genetically, men are predisposed to having more muscle. When you work out and build muscle, will not make you look like a man. Instead, it will actually make you look like a woman because your curves will be accentuated. Training for strength will certainly get you looking and feeling better as you build muscle. Other benefits include improved blood circulation and stronger bone health.

Chapter 3: Intermittent Fasting for Women

Intermittent fasting is believed to have different effects on women. There are numerous anecdotal effects of intermittent fasting reported in women, such as changes in the menstrual cycle, among other things. These changes are attributed to the fact that the female body is extremely sensitive to calorie restriction. In this chapter, we delve into the impact of intermittent fasting for women and offer tricks and tips to help you get started with your intermittent fasting journey.

Intermittent Fasting and the Female Body

The success of any diet, fitness, or nutrition program in women is dependent on a number of factors. These can be hormonal or biological. Women tend to experience more harmful risks and effects than men when starting out on intermittent fasting. These include the following:

Excessive fatigue. Muscle weakness and fatigue are the two most common side effects linked to a reduction in calorie intake in women. This is because these effects are magnified by the fact that the female body relies more on glucose than the stored fat for energy. Although these effects decrease over time and eventually disappear, they make the initial adaptation and transition to the fasting schedule to be more difficult in women than men, especially in the first few weeks.

Hormonal imbalance. Hormonal imbalances are common in women. However, with the introduction of intermittent fasting, this can evolve into more pressing issues relating to genetics. Some of the concerns during intermittent fasting include irregular menstruation; irregular length of your period or the strength of your flow, blemishes that are difficult to clear and changes in the skin tone.

Emotional instability. One of the issues that come with the fluctuating hormones during intermittent fasting is emotional instability. Most women report this, especially in the first two weeks to one month.

Overall, intermittent fasting is not all about health difficulties and concerns. The benefits of intermittent fasting for women far outweigh these challenges. Eventually, most women incorporate intermittent fasting to their daily lifestyle.

How Does Intermittent Fasting Benefit Women?

Women who have pre-existing heart conditions or are at risk of heart diseases and those with high cholesterol levels have credited intermittent fasting for improved health conditions. Of course, this is with the guidance of a medical professional. However, these are but few of the health benefits that women who have adopted intermittent fasting enjoy. Some of the positive health benefits of intermittent fasting for women are:

Increased insulin sensitivity. Intermittent fasting helps in reducing food cravings because it maintains normal levels of Ghrelin, the hunger hormone. Fasting is also pivotal in boosting autophagy, the natural mechanism through which the body cleanses itself by clearing and recycling old and unwanted cellular components for restoration and proper functioning of all the cellular processes. Intermittent fasting is effective in the treatment of Type 2 diabetes, as well as other conditions that are related to blood sugar. This is possible because of the increase in insulin production that is a result of fasting.

Decreased inflammation. Intermittent fasting reduces the risk of obesity in women because of the improvements in metabolic efficiency and body composition by burning visceral fat. Your blood pressure will also be lowered when you fast in addition to having greater control over any issues related to blood pressure. Another notable benefit of intermittent fasting in women has to do with the improved symptoms of auto-immune diseases like systemic lupus erythematosus (S.L.E), Crohn's disease, rheumatoid arthritis, and colitis, among others. Intermittent fasting contributes to lowering your blood pressure and give you greater control over any blood pressure related issues you may be having.

Improved functioning of the pancreas. Intermittent fasting causes an increase in the production of ketone bodies that enhance cognitive function and offer protection against neurological diseases such as Parkinson's disease, dementia, and Alzheimer's disease. The increase in insulin sensitivity that is triggered by fasting starve cancer cells, leaving them vulnerable to destruction. This is because cancer cells are receptive to insulin compared to the normal cells. You'll also have an increase in the production of HGH that is also known as the fitness hormone. This hormone is vital for promoting longevity and maintaining optimum health by burning fat pockets, promoting muscle development, and boosting metabolism.

Women who are in menopause also benefit from intermittent fasting by being able to lose the extra weight that comes with hormonal fluctuations. Besides, when you practice intermittent fasting, you'll be more stable emotionally and well empowered you to control your emotional impulses well.

Intermittent Fasting Risks for Women

Women taking part in intermittent fasting across the globe report that they experienced the same negative effects men felt. These include difficulty in concentrating or focusing throughout the day, dehydration and initial hunger pangs, muscle weakness, headaches, and initial loss of muscle tone.

In addition to these, women with a history of irregular periods have reported having symptoms of infertility as they continued with intermittent fasting over a considerable period of time. This is particularly common among women who experience dramatic fat loss, particularly in the first few weeks of their intermittent fasting schedule. The good news is that these changes are never permanent, so don't worry about it. In fact, periods usually return to normal, and fertility increases after stopping your intermittent fasting. Medical experts advise that women who are pregnant or are hoping to get pregnant soon should stay away from any intermittent fasting plan.

Intermittent Fasting for Post Menopause Women

Menopause is a time of transition in many ways for most women. In fact, chances are that you're going to deal with a lot of symptoms that come with it. From hot flashes, mood swings, cravings, sleep, confidence, temperature and weight gain, the challenges can be overwhelming. The average woman gains about four and a half pounds as she transitions into menopause in her 40s and another pound and a half in their 50s and 60s. this weight ends up accumulating around the abdomen, leaving you with what looks like a beer belly. While it's important to eat and keep your body well nourished, you also need to fast, and this is where intermittent fasting comes in.

Intermittent fasting helps in leveling out the hormonal imbalance, thus making your transition smooth. It's also an ideal way to keep your belly fat and body weight in check during this stage. All your hormones are interconnected; thus, your diet and eating patterns have an influence on your hormones. One study found that intermittent fasting can be a game-changer for women battling menopausal weight. Intermittent fasting can help you lose that fat. Menopausal women who practice intermittent fasting are likely to lose twice as much weight at premenopausal women because of better adherence to the diet.

Additionally, they are also likely to experience a 10-20% decrease in LDL cholesterol, a reduction in blood pressure, and a decrease in insulin resistance. It's important to keep in mind that women's bodies are more sensitive to changes during menopause. Therefore, it's important to build upon the length of your fasting period gradually. If intermittent fasting will aggravate your menopause symptoms, then it's advisable to stop immediately as this could be a sign that intermittent fasting is not for you.

Can All Women Practice Intermittent Fasting?

Intermittent fasting is not suitable for all women. However, it should be noted that it'll work perfectly for 99% of all women. However, this means that you've got to be more careful so that you don't get into health issues that are difficult to resolve. You're among the 1% of women who can't practice intermittent fasting if:

- You have sleep problems
- Your period is not regular/is suspended
- You're suffering from anxiety disorders
- Your hair is falling so fast
- You take long before you recover from injuries suffered during training
- Your body feels abnormally cold
- Your sex drive is low
- You're regularly experiencing mood swings

Intermittent fasting is also discouraged if you're pregnant. This is because the moment conception takes place, and a fetus is formed; it secures its nutrients regardless of the consequences this has on the mother. That is, it fights for survival as such it is inappropriate to practice intermittent fasting you're pregnant. In order to effectively practice intermittent fasting successfully, you'll need to listen to your body. Generally, you'll be able to tell if intermittent fasting is good for you once you get into it. Even then, this is not to say that you quit after two days because it's normal before your body gets used to staying for extended blocks of time without food. Most importantly, realize that intermittent fast will vary from one woman to the other, so don't put so much pressure on yourself.

Making Your Intermittent Fasting Plan to Succeed

When you start your intermittent fasting, you need to keep in mind that the results you anticipate to achieve are linked to having a long-term plan. This is because intermittent fasting is not designed to be an overnight success but a lifestyle. Therefore, you might as well consult a medical professional before getting into intermittent fasting. You'll need to ask a number of questions when creating your intermittent fasting schedule that includes the following:

Have you weighed the benefits and risks of intermittent fasting and decided what you can do for a smooth transition before starting?

Is your intermittent fasting plan realistic in relation to your health status as well as existing conditions and reaching your personal goals?

Have you spoken to a medical professional to ensure safe transition and consistency with your intermittent fasting plan?

Is intermittent fasting the best option for you?

Have you chosen the right intermittent fasting method that will meet my personal goals and needs?

What are my short term and long term health goals? Do you want to lose weight or you're seeking to achieve fitness goals.

When you have answers to all these questions, you can take the next steps to start intermittent fasting lifestyle. When you have a plan, you are able to get an idea of how your body will respond to extended fasting windows without having to worry about negative side effects such as excessive fatigue that come with switching abruptly. You'll do well to gather as much information about intermittent fasting, diets and working out to be sure about what works and what doesn't work. You'll also be able to get answers to all the questions you may be having about intermittent fasting either by searching the internet or speaking to a medical professional. When you're equipped with adequate information, it's easier to develop a routine that will deliver the results you desire, and you can comfortably stick to.

Find Your Motivation

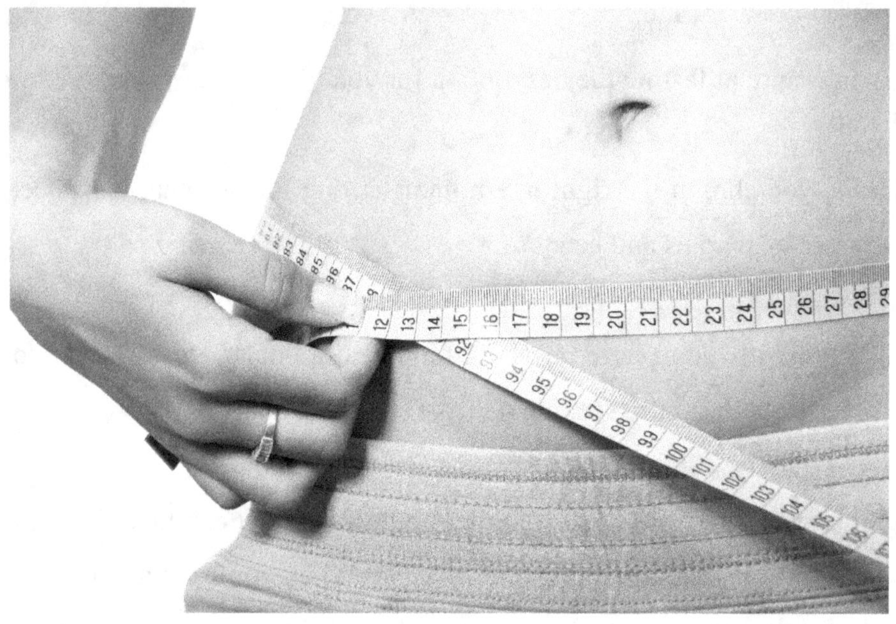

Diets and weight loss programs can be intimidating. Therefore, it's important to have a motivational goal that drives you. These goals need to be realistic because if they're not, it's unlikely that you'll stick to the plan. You must first understand why you're undertaking the challenge along with everything that comes with it. Remember, this health trend that is taking the health and fitness world by storm doesn't have to work for you just because it's working for everyone. Every kind of fitness or diet requires adaptability, determination, sacrifice, and focus. For these reasons, you need to clearly define what it is that is motivating you to start intermittent fasting. Setting goals is an excellent way of motivating yourself even on those days when temptation comes knocking or you have a trip coming up that is likely to interrupt your intermittent fasting schedule. When you know clearly what motivates you to start the fasting lifestyle, you can now set your expectations and goals for the routine you're committing yourself to follow. While it's difficult to know how your plan will work when you set goals, you have a reference point you can always come back to whenever you need to make the necessary adjustments to your schedule.

How to Get Your Body to Adapt to Fasting

If you have never tried the intermittent fasting lifestyle, you need to begin by i0ueasing your body into this pattern by restricting your calorie intake or even skipping meal daily for one week. This way, your body will not respond to intermittent fasting with shock because the body will take time to adjust and switch between fat burning and fat storing processes smoothly without shocking your digestive system. When you've seen your body's reaction to skipping meals and reduced calorie intake, you can fully embrace intermittent fasting that essentially means lessening more calories and eating lighter meals where you're not skipping. Minimizing your calorie intake before you begin intermittent fasting also lets you settle into the routine mentally.

That is, you'll be able to embrace and appreciate the role of intermittent fasting, making you have more control over your new habits and challenges that come with it.

Tips to Make Intermittent Fasting a Success

Make a gradual change. Like any other major lifestyle, fitness, or diet change, the best move you can ever make is to transition gradually. When you make sudden changes, your body gets into shock that could either clear over time or escalate into serious health concerns. This means that is you're getting into intermittent fasting as a quick fix for particular issues you may be facing then it's unlikely you'll get the results you want compared to someone who embraces it as a lifestyle change. When you transition gradually, you'll experience a number of benefits that include:

- Adequate time to monitor how your body is reacting to fasting as a regular part of your life so that you're able to make adjustments to ease any discomfort.

- You'll also find it easier to tweak, adjust, and fine-tune your intermittent fasting schedule to minimize the side effects and maximize the health benefits.

- You'll also mentally prepare for the social and physical changes you will undergo. Mental strength is the key to your success.

It's easy to get excited when you start your lifestyle journey; however, you must take time to understand the changes and feelings your body is going through with your personalized plan.

Choose a realistic intermittent fasting plan. One of the fundamental things you can do to make sure you succeed with intermittent fasting is to create a plan that fits into your schedule to that the transition is almost seamless. This will help you to follow the schedule for a prolonged time hence making it your lifestyle. While all the intermittent fasting plans can help you achieve your goals like weight loss so that you feel more confident, you've got to find one that suits you best.

Intermittent fasting must be approached with caution and where possible, with the health of a nutrition or health professional. Remember, just like any good thing intermittent fasting can end up in a tragedy when not addressed properly. So take your time to understand the whole concept in relation to your current health status before attempting it.

Chapter 4: Benefits of Intermittent Fasting

The popularity of intermittent fasting has been fueled by the benefits it promises. Although abstinence or withdrawal from food is a physical change, the rewards that come with it include psychological and spiritual wellbeing. In this section, we take a look at the benefits of incorporating intermittent fasting into your lifestyle. Here are some of the benefits that research has linked to intermittent fasting:

Intermittent Fasting May Extend Your Lifespan, Helping You Live Longer

Restricting calories is one of the reliable ways of increasing your lifespan significantly. Fasting also increases the lifespan of a number of organisms like worms and yeast. Although it's not explicit about cutting down your calories, intermittent fasting generally results in the reduction of your daily calorie consumption by between 10-30%. This results in improved insulin sensitivity, a reduction in free radical damage to cellular components namely DNA and proteins, lowering your blood pressure and heart rate, a reduction in the incidence of induced and spontaneous tumors and enhanced resistance to neurodegenerative diseases. In essence, intermittent fasting is an alternative to calorie restriction, which has a similar effect on the aging process and extension of your lifespan. When subjected to fasting, young rats had a longer lifespan exceeding their average lifespan by a couple of months. Fasting has the same effect in humans; when you embrace the intermittent fasting way of life, your body goes into stress due to calorie withdrawal. This is followed by the release of a range of chemicals that offer protection from the side effects of fasting. They also help in fighting anxiety and depression. Scientifically, it is believed that these chemicals help the body to develop increased resistance to stress that ultimately slows down the aging process while extending longevity.

Improved Heart Health

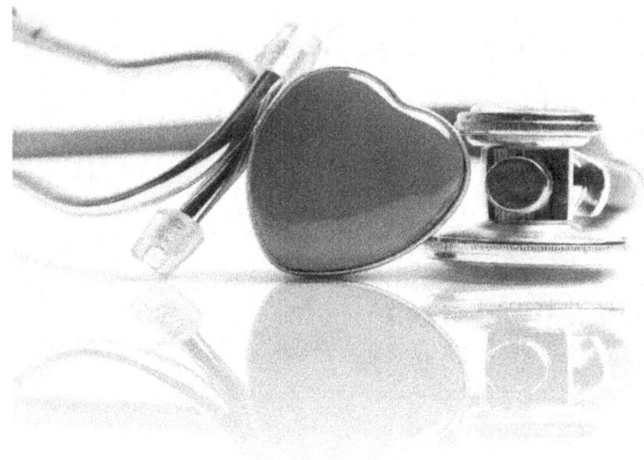

One study on the health benefits of intermittent fasting in participants who were non-obese found that there was a decrease in the levels of triglyceride in men and an increase in the good HDL cholesterol in women. This change was recorded within a span of 22 days, during which the participants took part in the study. This change was linked to a 4% degradation of body fat. These values improved significantly in obese people demonstrated by an average loss of 5.6kg over a period of eight weeks while on intermittent fasting. This was translated in a 21% drop in cholesterol levels, a 32% decrease in triglycerides, and a 25% drop in LDL cholesterol levels.

Similarly, the systolic blood pressure dropped from 124 mmHg to 116 mmHg. Apart from the reduction of body weight, intermittent fasting also induces stress resistance that has a cardioprotective effect. Studies conducted in mice also show that in the event of a heart attack, the area that is affected is half times smaller in those mice that were fasting than in the normally fed mice. Additionally, in cardiac infarction, four times fewer heart muscles died when the mice were fed intermittently.

Intermittent Fasting Reduces the Risk of Cancer

Intermittent fasting has been found to slow down the development and progression of malignant tumors. Rats transplanted with a cancer cell line were subjected to intermittent fasting, and the result is that they survived for a longer period than their counterparts that were free-fed. After ten days, 50% of the rats that were on intermittent fasting were still alive, while only 12.5% of those in the control group were alive. Another study in middle-aged rats that were subjected to intermittent fasting and observed for a period of four months saw a reduced incidence of lymphoma. While 30% of the mice in the control group became ill while none of the rats on intermittent fasting became cancerous. Intermittent fasting also saw a reduction in the development of pre-neoplastic liver injury and liver nodules that are caused by carcinogenic substances. The rats that ate intermittently also had better antioxidant activity resulting in reduced development of harmful free radicals in the mitochondria. It's worth noting that this antitumor effect is not a result of calorie reduction since both groups consumed the same number of calories.

Improved Brain Power

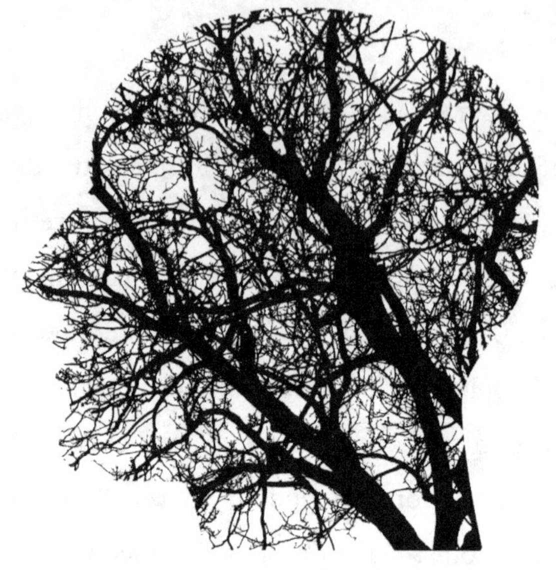

Intermittent fasting enhances neuronal functionality that often decreases with the advancement of age. As you grow old, your dendritic spines that are small membranous protrusions from the neuron of a dendrite will decrease. Dendritic spines have a crucial role in the transfer of information between nerve cells. However, these spines reduce with age, thus affecting the efficiency of neural processes adversely. Intermittent fasting will prevent the reduction of the dendritic spines density. Rats that were on a normal diet had a 38% decline in the number of dendritic spines.

On the contrary, the rats that were on intermittent fasting had a near negligible difference in a young rat that after 24 hours. If anything, the rats had improved learning abilities. The calorie reduction that is triggered by intermittent fasting increases the process of neurogenesis, which is essentially the formation of new brain cells, while also protecting the neurons from dying. Furthermore, it also stimulates the production of Brain-Derived Neurotropic Factor (BDNF), which is a protein that is linked to the increase in the process of neurogenesis. This slows down the neuron degenerations and eventually aging. The effect on neurogenesis also promotes functional recovery as well as the healing of injuries to the spinal cord in animals even when intermittent fasting is introduced before or after the injury.

Intermittent Fasting Can Help You Lose Weight and Belly Fat

Intermittent fasting can drive weight loss because it lowers insulin levels. During fasting, your body will not have access to glucose for energy. Instead, when you're in the fasted state, your body breaks down carbohydrates to glucose that the cells use for energy or convert it into fat and store. Insulin is the hormone that enables cells to take in glucose. Your insulin level is likely to begin decreasing when you stop consuming food. This drop in insulin level causes cells to tap into the glucose stores for energy. When you fast repeatedly, you'll begin to experience weight loss. This is unlike diets that are usually designed to be implemented over a short period, so once you get back to your normal diet, you begin gaining weight again. With intermittent fasting, you can maintain the change in weight loss for some time because it's easy to stick to and doesn't require a special meal plan. This means you can still eat your favorite food as long as you schedule your meals properly and maintain a longer fasting window. Intermittent fasting will induce ketosis and autophagy that eventually reduce fat reserves.

Intermittent Fasting Can Help in the Prevention of Diseases

It's natural for sick animals to stop eating while recovering. This also applies to humans. Intermittent fasting is the key to overall wellbeing because it helps in the prevention of a number of medical conditions and diseases. A number of studies have found the benefits of intermittent on overall health. More specifically, a study in the World Journal of Diabetes has shown that patients who have type 2 diabetes and are on a short term intermittent fasting experience a reduction in their body weight along with better post-meal glucose variability. Other related benefits include reduced blood pressure, reduced inflammation, better glucose circulation, and lipid levels that can lead to a reduced risk of neurological and cardiovascular diseases. Beyond all the specific diseases and illnesses, fasting offers a range of benefits that go to boost the immune system, thus protecting you from all kinds of potential illnesses.

Intermittent Fasting Helps in Improving Physical Fitness

Apart from mental performance, intermittent fasting also helps in improving physical performance. When you have a short feeding window and an extended fasting period, you'll have proper digestion with the result being healthy and proportional daily food and calorie intake. As you get used to this plan, it's unlikely that you will experience hunger. Intermittent fasting enhances your metabolism making your body to effectively run on energy from glucose and fats.

Intermittent Fasting Lowers the Risk of Type 2 Diabetes

According to CDC, at least 84.1 million people in the U.S. have pre-diabetes which when left uncontrolled can result in the type 2 diabetes. Intermittent fasting is pivotal in lowering/preventing the risk of type 2 diabetes. This is based on the fact that it helps in weight loss; hence, can potentially influence various other factors that contribute to a high risk of diabetes. For instance, when you lose weight, you'll become insulin sensitive. A paper published in the Translational research concluded that there's enough evidence pointing to the role influence of intermittent fasting on lowering insulin levels and blood glucose. According to the paper, intermittent fasting is promising for weight loss and reduction of diabetes. There was a noticeable decrease in markers of diabetes, like insulin sensitivity in Obese and overweight adults. Thus, intermittent fasting could lower the risk of type 2 diabetes in this group of people because it requires the body to produce insulin less often. Intermittent fasting is critical in the restoration of insulin secretion while promoting the generation of insulin-producing pancreatic beta cells.

Intermittent Fasting Helps to Sync Circadian Rhythms and Fight off Metabolic Diseases

The circadian rhythm that is commonly referred to as the sleep/wake cycle is a natural and internal system that is designed to regulate feelings of wakefulness and sleepiness over a period of 24-hours. Research has shown that one of the benefits of practicing intermittent fasting is that the body is able to stick to its natural circadian rhythm that is good for metabolism. Eating certain foods before bed has been linked to sleep disturbances and weight gain, especially if it causes acid reflux. This is because insulin sensitivity is usually high during the day and quite low at night. This means that your body is likely to store most of the glucose consumed at night, resulting in weight gain. It is important that you go to bed and sleep early to give the body ample time to repair itself.

Intermittent Fasting May Help in Prevention of Alzheimer's disease

Alzheimer's disease is the most common neurodegenerative disease in the world. Since there's no cure for this disease, prevention of the same is critical. A study conducted in rats showed that practicing intermittent fasting could delay the development of Alzheimer's disease. In cases where the disease is already existing, intermittent fasting lessens its severity. A number of reports corroborate with this as they suggest that a lifestyle intervention that includes fasting on the short term will significantly improve the symptoms of Alzheimer's disease in 9 out of 10 patients. Studies conducted on animals suggest that fasting can protect against other neurodegenerative diseases that include Huntington's and Parkinson's disease. Even then, more studies need to be done in humans.

Intermittent Fasting for an Improved Physical Fitness

Intermittent fasting has an influence on your digestive system. When you have a small window within which to feed, you encourage proper digestion of food. Consequently, you encourage proportional and healthy daily intake of calories and food. As you get used to this routine, you'll bare experience hunger. One of the common misconceptions about this pattern of eating is that it slows down metabolism. Intermittent fasting enhances your metabolism by making it more flexible because the body now has the ability to run on glucose or fat for energy effectively. This means that intermittent fasting enhances metabolism.

Intermittent Fasting Leads to Increased Energy

While it's highly likely that you'll feel lethargic during the first few days into intermittent fasting, you'll not always have lowered energy levels. In fact, the opposite is true. When you fast, your body stops relying on glucose from the food you eat and shifts focus on the fat stores. This is not only a great source of energy, but it also leaves you feeling energized for extended periods.

Intermittent Fasting Helps in Enhancing Body Building

Having a small feeding window translates to fewer meals meaning you need to concentrate your daily calorie intake in 1-2 consistent meals. Most bodybuilders find this approach to be great compared to having the same calorie consumption distributed in 5 to 6 different meals spread out through the day. While it's believed that your body requires a certain amount of proteins to maintain your muscle mass, it's important to keep in mind that you can also maintain muscle mass through intermittent fasting. This is backed by the increase in the growth hormone after 48 hours of fasting that makes it easy to maintain muscle mass without eating proteins or taking protein shakes.

Promotes the Production of the Neuron Growth Hormone

During intermittent fasting, your body will start operating on a cycle that is based on ketones. Consequently, you'll experience and increased the production of the brain-derived-neurotropic factor (BDNF). This is a protein that promotes neuron growth within the brain. It also protects these neurons from any other form of damage.

Intermittent Fasting Offers Therapeutic Benefits

The benefits of intermittent fasting are not only physical but also spiritual and psychological. Physical benefits like curing diabetes and reduction of seizures relating to brain damage or even improving symptoms of arthritis go hand in hand with spiritual benefits for which fasting is practiced across different religions all over the globe. On the psychological aspect, intermittent fasting requires you to exercise control and will power over your feelings and body. Achieving this absolute control over your mind and power is a great psychological effect. Ignoring hunger and exercising restrain from eating over an extended period will have a powerful psychological point of view.

Intermittent Fasting Can Reduce Oxidative Stress and Inflammation

Oxidative stress is one of the stages of many chronic disease and aging. It involves numerous molecules referred to as free radicals that react with other useful molecules and damage them. A number of studies have shown that intermittent fasting is a great way to enhance the body's resistance to oxidative stress. Moreover, intermittent fasting can also help in fighting inflammation that is a major driver of a majority of diseases.

Intermittent Fasting Changes the Function of Cells, Genes, and Hormones

Failure to eat for a long period initiates a number of processes in the body. Among the processes are cellular repair processes and changes in your hormonal levels aimed at making the stored body fat more accessible as a source of energy. Some of the common changes that will occur include a drop in insulin levels that leads to fat burning, your growth hormone levels may also increase to trigger further fat burning and muscle gain. The body also induces cellular repair processes like removal of waste material from the cells. There are also other beneficial changes in molecules and genes that relate to protection against disease and longevity.

Intermittent Fasting Induces Various Cellular Processes

You are made up of cells. That is, cells are the building blocks of life with the body comprising of over trillions of cells. These cells keep you alive through a process of regeneration. During fasting, your body initiates a cellular cell regeneration process that is referred to as autophagy. This process involves breaking down cells as well as metabolize of dysfunctional and broken proteins that tend to build up within the cell with time.

Side Effects of Intermittent Fasting

Although intermittent fasting comes with multiple health and wellness benefits, it's also important to highlight the fact that it can also have side effects. This will vary from individual to the other. Among the common side effects that you can experience include the following:

Short term downsides. These generally refer to the body's reaction to the withdrawal or abstinence of food. The common short-lived but adverse effects of practicing intermittent fasting include headaches, dizziness, weakness, outbursts, gout, low blood pressure, and gall stones.

Poor weight management. For most people who embrace intermittent fasting for weight loss, it can be difficult to maintain a healthy weight. This is because of cravings for some calories after an extended period of fasting that eventually counteract the progress made during fasting.

Long term downsides. When you fast for prolonged periods of time, your immune system could be weakened, thus affecting your vital organs that include the liver and kidneys. When you stay for a long period without eating, you might end up being malnourished which, when not checked, can eventually lead to untimely death because your energy reserve is completely depleted.

Hunger. This is a common side effect of abstaining from food for extended periods of time. When you're used to eating several times a day, your body expects food at certain times. The hunger hormone, ghrelin, peaks at breakfast, lunch, and dinner. However, this doesn't last for long as it eases up as you get used to the intermittent fasting routine. In fact, with the time, you'll feel less hungry when fasting. You can also drink black tea and coffee to curb hunger. Most importantly, make sure you keep yourself busy, get enough sleep, and avoid strenuous workouts because they can increase hunger.

Cravings. When you go for extended periods without eating, you'll most likely think about eating. This is when you begin to have cravings, especially for sweets or processed carbohydrates because your body needs glucose.

Headaches. When you start fasting intermittently, you'll experience headaches. This is often linked to dehydration. Therefore, make sure that you drink up enough water and other non-caloric fluids during both feeding and fasting window.

Constipation, bloating, and heartburn. Your stomach usually produces acid to aid digestion. As such, when you're not eating, you could experience heartburn. This may result in mild discomfort to frequent burping. Make sure you take adequate water and avoid spicy and greasy foods that can worsen your heartburn.

Low energy. When you fast, your body is deprived of its source of energy. Your energy levels will be low. Subsequently, you will feel a little sluggish. To cope with this feeling, keep your day relaxed and avoid exerting the least amount of energy. At this point, you might want to take a break from workouts.

Irritability. When your blood sugars levels drop due to intermittent fasting, you can start feeling cranky. You can deal with this by avoiding people or situations that can annoy you and focus on those things that uplift your spirit and make you feel happy.

Feeling cold. Cold toes and fingers are common when you're fasting.

This is because your blood flows to your fat stores increase. When your blood sugar decreases, you become more sensitive to feeling cold.

Advantages and Disadvantages of Intermittent Fasting

There are two sides to every good thing. Likewise, intermittent fasting has both advantages and disadvantages. This section takes a look at both the pros and cons of practicing the intermittent fasting lifestyle:

Advantages of Intermittent Fasting

It's flexible. One good thing about intermittent fasting is that you get to choose a plan that suits your lifestyle. This means that you get to fast at your convenience as long as you're achieving the defined hours of fasting/feasting depending on your plan.

Intermittent fasting saves you time. When you start fasting, you'll be surprised at how much time you'll save that you'll otherwise have spent in shopping for groceries and preparing meals. You can spend this time doing other productive activities. Besides, the freedom this gives you is liberating.

You save on grocery bills. Skipping a single meal a couple of times a week or month can save you a lot of money. Intermittent fasting will definitely reduce the amount of money you spent on grocery bills and save you money.

It's easy to follow. Unlike other weight-loss diets, intermittent fasting doesn't require you to track the food you eat or even calculate the ratios and percentages of the nutrients you're consuming. Furthermore, you don't have to purchase expensive ingredients or even come up with costly meal plans. You can do it with what you have.

Disadvantages of Intermittent Fasting

It takes time to settle into the program. If you're used to snacking or eating every few hours, adjusting into intermittent fasting plan. In fact, the first few weeks will be the hardest. At first, hunger pangs can be uncomfortable and painful in extreme cases.

Lethargy. Although it doesn't last for long, intermittent fasting will leave you feeling lethargic. This can make it difficult to work or even concentrate, especially in the workplace. However, you can address this by adjusting your schedule so that your eating window falls within the time you'll be working.

Hormonal imbalance in women. In most cases, dietary changes will impact your hormonal balance because it influences the production of hormones. You can counter this by easing into the diet, gradually giving your body ample time to adjust accordingly.

You can go overboard with fasting. When you embrace intermittent fasting, you might end up going overboard, especially if you want to achieve results faster. This can leave you nutrient-deprived, giving rise to a myriad of health complications.

You'll have the temptation to overeat upon breaking your fast. It's common to have the urge to eat more food when you break your fast. This is particularly common during the first few weeks and is counterproductive. Therefore, you need to train yourself mentally to restrict your consumption of food to a normal amount.

Chapter 5: Intermittent Fasting and Autophagy

Intermittent fasting and autophagy are intertwined. In fact, autophagy ranks high among weight loss methods, just like intermittent fasting. Most people who've embraced it give a guarantee that autophagy is indeed a life changer. So what then is autophagy? The term autophagy is derived from two words; 'auto' meaning self and 'phagein' meaning to engulf. Thus, autophagy is the process where harmful microbes, damaged cell organelles, and other components that are unwanted in the body are engulfed. This process aims at eliminating these components, regenerate new cells, and detoxify the body.

History of Autophagy

The term autophagy was first coined by Christian de Duve, a Belgian scientist during his study of lysosomes and the glucagon's role in cell degeneration. Researchers began studying cellular autophagy by closely looking at cellular autophagy. The only challenge then is that there was little information about the importance of this process to the human body and overall wellbeing. It wasn't until 1983 that Yoshinori Ohsumi made a discovery of the gene that is important in the regulation of autophagy in yeast. This discovery was a huge milestone because he discovered that yeast cells that lacked those genes didn't go through autophagy. Consequently, these cells couldn't repair themselves. Ohsumi went on to be awarded a Nobel Prize for this discovery in 2016.

The major takeaways from the discovery Ohsumi made are how cells respond to nutrient deficiency, an increase in stress levels, cellular injuries and deprivation of energy through an increased rate of cellular autophagy or the stress response mode. However, when the stress is eliminated, the autophagy process goes back to maintenance mode that is the regular rate. More studies need to be done to fully understand this process of engulfment and its relation to aging while relating the effect of the same on stress levels. Existing evidence suggests that the process that enhances autophagy will also see an extension of your lifespan. The belief here is that cell aging occurs where unwanted cellular components begin accumulating, yet they are not removed properly. Because of its ability to remove damaged cell materials, autophagy is believed to slow down the aging process. For this reason, scientists are seeking to do further studies to extend life expectancy.

The Autophagy Process

There are three ways through which autophagy can occur; microautophagy, macroautophagy, and sweets autophagy. All these involve transportation of cellular waste to lysosomes where it's broken down before recycling.

Microautophagy. When microautophagy occurs, cellular wastes that are meant to be digested is mopped by lysosomes either by developing cellular protrusions or inward folding of a section of the lysosomal membrane.

Macroautophagy. During macroautophagy, all the waste material within a cell is transported through an autophagosome, a double membrane-bound vesicle, to the lysosome. The autophagosome fuses with the lysosome emptying all its content making room for waste materials to be processed.

Chaperone mediated autophagy. During this process, the cell uses chaperone proteins like Hsc-70 that are on the lysosomal membrane. These proteins bind to protein molecules that are unwanted in the cell to form a substrate/chaperone complex. It's this molecule that eventually attaches with lysosome wall allowing the protein molecules to enter into the lysosome where it disintegrates.

All three autophagy processes involve selective and non-selective degradation methods that are dependent on the organelles or molecules that require breaking down or recycling. Ultimately, all the cellular components that must be degraded are collected from the lysosome before converting to micro molecules like nucleotides, glucose, fatty acids, and amino acids. The micro molecules are later reused by the cell in the formation of larger molecules as well as new organelles. Thus, these autophagy processes rejuvenate the body's cells, leaving you feeling healthier, younger, and better.

Relationship between Autophagy and Apoptosis

Apoptosis refers to the programmed death of a cell that happens as part of the normal activities of the cell. Cell death is necessary for there to be a balance between healthy and good cells and those that are senescent. How is this process related to autophagy? Understanding the relationship between apoptosis and autophagy could be the solution to the management and treatment of various diseases that include Alzheimer's disease because of the ability of both processes to regulate cell death.

Activating Autophagy

Autophagy doesn't take place as soon as you begin your intermittent fasting schedule. It takes time. It's activated by nutrient deprivation. The number of factors determines when autophagy will set in. From your state of health to body fat percentage and activity levels.

Most importantly, it's dependent on the amount of effort you're willing to put in to get your body to attain autophagy. But first, what stops autophagy? When the level of various body nutrients like calories, glucose, and amino acids are low, there's a need for autophagy. This is because the body is not motivated to seek energy from fat stores and body tissues. However, this can happen under the right conditions. When the body nutrients are sufficient, a signal is received by mTOR and AMPK. The cells then decide whether to promote growth or switch to intermittent fasting. Other factors that determine what will happen are growth factors like IGF – 1, insulin, and mechanical muscle stimuli.

Generally, a 48-72 hour fast is recommended to activate autophagy. This is also the duration of time it takes for ketosis to take place when the body produces ketones. Ultimately, there's no accurate way of measuring the autophagy rate in humans. Even then, it can be estimated by taking into account the glucose ketone index and the insulin to glucose ratio. When this ratio is low, a breakdown of nutrients, gluconeogenesis, fat oxidations, and ketogenesis take place. The duration it'll take for the autophagy process to set in will depend on your body nutrients, the presence of nutrients in your ketones, glucose, and amino acids. Thus, if your body is conditioned not to consume excessive protein and fat daily, it will be faster to get into autophagy compared to someone that has to burn a lot more calories initially.

Autophagy and Anti-Aging Effects?

The presence of cellular waste and non-functional components within the cell degrades your health and the quality of life, making you look older than you are. The result of this is an increase in the elimination of the aging cells. This is where autophagy comes in handy because it helps in slowing down the aging mechanism so that you look healthier and younger for a long time.

Benefits of Autophagy

Although important, metabolic activities cause cellular damage to the human body over time. The rate at which cellular damage occurs increases with age due to poor diet, stress, and exposure to radiation, among other factors. When autophagy takes place, the damaged and old cells that are inactive are eliminated from the body. This process is also important in purging the body of infection-causing pathogens. The result of this is that you get to experience a number of health benefits that include the following:

Extension of the average lifespan. Although there are numerous methods and techniques that guarantee the improvement of health, among other benefits, autophagy is the most outstanding of them all. Cells are the building blocks of life; therefore, autophagy will help in eliminating waste materials from these blocks. The removal of toxic substances from the body enhances metabolic efficiency of the cells as they become healthy. Cellular degeneration and regeneration processes triggered by autophagy will help you to stay youthful than you actually are. This is particularly helpful for your skin that is exposed to pollutants and harsh elements, causing wrinkles and a decline in the quality of your skin.

Decreases the risk of cell death. In some cases, the cells in your body can degrade beyond the point of replacement or regeneration resulting in cell death, also known as apoptosis. This is bad because the cells that are spared during apoptosis are irreparable meaning that when you lose them, you'll lose them for a lifetime. Autophagy prevents this hence, also preventing diseases that are linked with cell death.

Regulates inflammation. You can reduce or boost your immune response with autophagy by promoting and preventing inflammation.

When there's a dangerous invader, autophagy will boost inflammation by signaling the immune system to attack. It can decrease inflammation by getting rid of those signals that cause it.

Helps the body to deal with stress. Autophagy can help in the treatment and prevention of psychiatric diseases like schizophrenia and depression.

Improvement in body metabolism. Autophagy plays a crucial role in boosting your metabolism. It achieves this by regenerating and replacing the important cells related to metabolism like mitochondria. Autophagy also improves your digestive system by promoting good metabolism. This has an effect on muscle performance by promoting muscle mass development and cell growth. This also prevents stress relating to muscle injuries.

Improves your skin. Your skin is the largest organ in the body yet most susceptible to damages from adverse weather, air pollutions, heat, light, sunshine, and chemicals, among other things. These make the skin cells to age faster. Autophagy comes in to help in replacing new cells as well as repairing old ones. This is great because the skin cells help in getting rid of bacteria that infiltrate the body; thus, you have to energize them to become active.

Protection of neurodegenerative disorders. Autophagy will help in preventing the onset of degenerative diseases like Parkinson's disease, dementia, and Alzheimer's disease. These diseases thrive when there's an accumulation of toxic and old neurons that pile up in certain areas of your brain before spreading to the surrounding areas. Thus, autophagy comes in to replace parts of the useless neuron parts and before regenerating new ones.

Strengthens immunity system. Autophagy will keep your body's immunity in form by protecting you from potential infections by removing toxins from within the cells. It also destroys harmful microbes. It does so by promoting inflammation on cells and fighting diseases. Cellular inflammation enhances the cells immune system whenever there is an attack from different diseases. Autophagy induces this inflammation by making cell proteins to work more actively by starving them of nutrition. This instigates the requisite immune response to fight infections and diseases.

Combating infectious diseases. Autophagy can help in spring the immune system into action. It can get rid of some microbes from the body cells like Mycobacterium tuberculosis or the deadly viruses like HIV. Autophagy takes care of the toxins that come about due to the infections.

Prevents the onset of cancer. Autophagy has received widespread attention from the medical world because of its preventive capabilities on cancer. Autophagy has been found to prevent or inhibit the growth of early-stage cancer. Cancer is a result of cellular disorders and autophagy comes in to prevent these disorders by regulating damage response that is caused by DNA, promoting cellular inflammation, and regulating genome instability.

Negative Side Effects of Autophagy

Despite the numerous benefits that autophagy offers, it also comes with negative side effects. While autophagy regulates immunity and inflammation, some bacteria like Bartonella, Coxiella, and Brucella divide and multiply through this process. Thus, you could end up with an overgrowth of bacteria. Recent studies have found that the ATG6/BECN1 autophagy gene that is important in suppressing tumors in cancer cells is no longer that impactful. The study further suggests that the self-replicating effect of these process could promote the multiplication of cancer cells. The self-eating process is likely to make tumor cells resilient, causing them to survive against environmental stressors that could make them survive starvation and chemotherapy. This makes autophagy a better preventive measure than a treatment plan for cancer.

Common Autophagy Mistakes to Avoid

Attempting to get your body into autophagy can result in some mistakes that can be counterproductive to your efforts. Knowing these errors will help you to avoid them so that you stay on the right path and achieve the results you desire. Since you now know that the best way to activate autophagy is through intermittent fasting here are some of the common mistakes you need to avoid to activate autophagy:

Ending your fasting window too soon. You'll need to fast for at least 3 to five days before your body can go into the state of autophagy. Even then, this duration is not the same because some people will attain it early while others will attain it much later. This is because the duration it takes before autophagy is activated is determined by an individual as well as the balance between your AMPK and mTOR. While some people are able to attain autophagy with a 16 hour fast, this is not a very common occurrence because fasting doesn't begin the moment you stop eating. Your body has to digest the nutrients first meaning you need about 10 hours in the post-absorptive state. This means that your body only gets into the fasted state after about 6 hours after eating.

A discrepancy in your Circadian Rhythm. You can rarely achieve autophagy if you're not getting adequate sleep. Growth hormone also occurs in this manner and are released between 11 pm and 2am. This means that if you desire to get the most out of autophagy, you need to go to bed early and get adequate restful sleep early enough because it is then that major repair takes place. You get real benefits of autophagy during sleep. In fact, calorie restriction and the length of your fast won't matter if you're getting inadequate sleep.

Taking artificial sweeteners. Although some artificial sweeteners claim to have zero calories, they can sometimes raise your insulin level resulting in the release of insulin by the gut. Generally, when you think of, see or smell food, your appetite levels rise. This is followed by a release of insulin along with gastric juices before you eat. This food sensation prepares your digestive system ready for the release of insulin. Some of the common artificial sweeteners that are known to raise the blood sugar and insulin levels include saccharin, sucralose, and aspartame. Others that are also suspected to increase insulin levels are erythritol and stevia. The important thing is knowing how these sweeteners affect you and avoiding them.

Consuming fatty coffee. Although fats will not raise your level of insulin, as carbs and proteins do, they, on the other hand, raise your mTOR levels, thus putting your body in the feasting state. However, you can activate chaperone-mediated autophagy and macroautophagy that is induced by excessive hunger by adding boosting fats like MCT oil into your coffee. The only challenge with this is that when the fat is in excess, it'll enhance your insulin level effectively raising your mTOR, thus breaking the fast. For this reason, it is recommended that you only put a single spoon of ketone boosting fats. You can stay away from all sources of calories altogether to be sure that you're safe. In fact, avoid MCT oil in your coffee unless you're extending your fast and need an energy boost.

You supplement with calories. You can easily break your fast with supplements that come with extra calories and sugar. Although most supplements are safe to use, you must check their calorie content or even avoid too many supplements because they'll pile up excess calories enough to break your fast. This is why it's usually advisable to avoid calories during fasting.

Eating too little food nutrients. It's wrong to fast for extended periods and not eat enough food nutrients when the time to feast comes. This jeopardizes your overall health because fasting decreases the amount the food nutrients that the body receives. This makes it necessary for you to include sufficient food nutrients in your meals. Make sure that you concentrate on foods that are nutrient-dense such as wild fish, pastured eggs, beef, herbs, organ meats, low carb berries, vegetables, spices, and fruits. Fast foods don't give you the essential micronutrients that you need.

Failure to exercise. While it's true that fasting will activate autophagy, it's not the only thing but just a part of the equation. Thus, you must make sure you get adequate nutrition, sleep, and exercise. This means that when you're fasting, make sure you include low impact exercise to your regime. Exercise, along with restricted training, is a sure way of inducing autophagy and getting all the related benefits. When you fast without exercising, you will not reach your maximum health potential.

Common Misconceptions About Autophagy

As more and more people continue to embrace intermittent fasting because of its health benefits, so has there been a rise in speculations and misconceptions about the concept of autophagy. The truth is that while it is connected to intermittent fasting, autophagy is a broad concept with so many things to learn. This chapter seeks to debunk some of the myths about autophagy. Some of the misconceptions include the following:

More autophagy is better. You need to fast for at least three days before you can begin to experience the significance of autophagy. By the time you're getting to your third day of fasting, you will begin to fully experience the benefits of autophagy and fasting in general. This is because, during this time, you get to energize your body so that it fights of tumors and cancer cells as well as boost the production of stem cells. Despite these benefits, it doesn't then follow that more autophagy is the best. In fact, prolonged autophagy has its own side effects that include the following:

-Tumor cells can develop tough skin that will eventually make them resilient and tough. Consequently, they could even become resistant to treatment.

-Autophagy can sometimes offer a conducive environment for some parasites like bacteria and brucella to reproduce.

-Excessive autophagy comes with the risk of sarcopenia and muscle wasting that eventually affect longevity.

-While the ATG6/BECN1 is an essential autophagy gene that encodes the Beclin1 protein and is also critical to the reduction of cancer cells. However, excessive autophagy can instead feed the cancer cells, thus giving them energy and strength to survive.

The fact that autophagy is incredible is not in dispute. However, it becomes counterproductive when your body is in the autophagy state all the time that you no longer tap into the benefits. Instead, you'll end up with some health repercussions and health hazards that are unwanted. The best way to get the most from autophagy is by inducing it intermittently through successive durations of fasting and feasting. This is far much beneficial than constantly being in autophagy.

You can activate autophagy with a 24 hour fast. You cannot activate autophagy with a 24 hour fast. The best way to initiate autophagy within a short period is by combining fasting with a high-intensity exercise regimen. This means that even a 16-hour fast is not enough to trigger autophagy. The reason is simple; your body doesn't get into the fasted state immediately you abstain from eating. This is because your body will still ingest food nutrients from the food and draw its energy from it.

Consequently, your body will be in a post-absorptive state of metabolism for a couple of hours after your last fast. Remember that it takes some time before some foods like fibers, vegetables, fat, and proteins are properly digested. This means that your body is in the fed state and dependent on the calories you consumed. Because of this, your body will only get into the fasted state after about 5 to 6 hours of refraining from eating. This means that if you take your last meal of the day at 8 pm, you will not begin to feel the real physiological effect of your fast until 1 am. This means that if you're going to be on a 16 hour fast, you will actually have fasted for 12 hours, which is shorter to trigger autophagy. However, you'll still be able to experience the other benefits of intermittent fastings, such as fat burning and reduced inflammation.

Autophagy equals starvation. It's largely assumed that autophagy will make you starve. This is far from reality. When you stay away from food for so many hours in order to accomplish autophagy, this is different from starvation. When you're starved, you'll barely have the energy to engage in your day to day activities. But when you fast, you'll still have energy. Besides, intermittent fasting will not deprive your body of energy because:

The autophagy process breaks down old cells and proteins that serve as an additional source of protein when you're not feeding. When you fast, the body will rely on other body components for energy.

The body stores all the unused energy in the form of fats. When there's scarcity, it turns to this reserve for energy. These stored fats can keep you going for the time when you'll not be eating.

After a couple of days of fasting, your body will go into ketosis. That is, the normal metabolism process is suspended because there's no new food consumption. At this point, the body goes into a process where it only relies on ketones and stored fat for energy to power the muscle and brain.

Basal autophagy and longevity will improve through basal autophagy. This is one of the keys to a long life that is linked to restricting calories.

As you can see, the process of autophagy and intermittent fasting is not the same as starvation. During these processes, the body undergoes self-renewal and healing, which doesn't happen when the body is in the fasting state.

Autophagy eats up loose skin. It's a common myth that autophagy will cause loose skin to shrink, thereby tightening it after you've lost weight. There's no truth in this belief. Instead, studies have shown that autophagy is crucial to making people look younger by slowing down the skin's aging process. This means that autophagy can slow down the aging process that is prominently revealed in the skin. Even then, autophagy will not take away the wrinkles, and loose skin; rather, it fosters the process that keeps the skin elastic and healthy, making it tighten faster. Intermittent fasting along with autophagy will help in guarding against extreme loose skin when you go lose considerable weight. This means that you may have to deal with having loose skin when you shed off excess body fat. Even then, the good news is that autophagy will cause the skin to fit perfectly on your new body because of its role in the production of collagen and fibroblast.

Autophagy contributes to building muscle. Your body requires calories to be able to build muscle. Because of this, it is impossible to build muscle when you're in the fasted state without an additional source of energy. In particular, proteins are essential for building muscle since it requires an essential process that is known as muscle protein synthesis. When you fast, you limit your protein intake effectively switching your body in a catabolic state that breaks it down as opposed to the anabolic state that lets it grow.

Moreover, autophagy also contributes to the breaking down of old proteins that are floating around the body cells. This may be a functional ingredient in muscle protein synthesis. However, the problem is that some essential amino acids that are important for muscle protein synthesis like leucine will be missing. This is why it's rare to find someone who is overweight to begin building muscle and losing body fat when they begin resistance training.

Fat doesn't stop autophagy. Although the fat will not spike your insulin levels the way carbs and proteins do, it transitions your body into the fed state. Ketosis will foster the process of macroautophagy within the brain by the enhancement of Sirt 1. Chaperone-mediated autophagy will also get activated with ketone bodies in a manner that works on individual substrates as well as amino acids. When you fast while you're on a ketogenic diet, your beta-hydroxybutyrate and ketone levels increase. However, mTor will not respond to glucose and amino acids but also other available calories. This means that any excess energy will suppress the process of autophagy. Although fat doesn't entirely stop the process of autophagy, it slows it down to a certain level. Overall, the amount of fat you've consumes will determine if fat prevents the autophagy process of not. Keep in mind that as little as a single tablespoon of MCT oil is enough to enhance chaperone-mediated autophagy.

Drinking coffee hinders autophagy. Taking unsweetened coffee doesn't break your fast of work against autophagy. Instead, coffee is important in inducing autophagy and ketosis. Coffee has polyphenol, a compound that is known to promote the process of autophagy. Caffeine also lets your body enjoy lipolysis, a process that burns fat, boosts AMPK, improves ketones, and reduces insulin. Ultimately, make sure that you take your coffee unsweetened and without cream or milk because these will increase your insulin level hence stopping the benefits of your fast.

Consuming meat will hinder the autophagy process. Most people believe that meats, as well as diets that are high in protein, will work against the process of autophagy and that they cause you to age quickly. When you want to understand autophagy and put it in perspective, the number of times that you'll eat is crucial. When you don't fast for more than 24 hours, and you consume three meals, then you're unlikely to achieve autophagy. The best way to attain autophagy is through intermittent fasting that is combined with calorie restriction when you're on a carnivorous diet. Remember, carbs and insulin do not help the autophagy process.

Eating fruits doesn't break autophagy. Naturally, fruits contain fructose that is easily digested by the liver before being stored as liver glycogen. However, when in excess the fructose is converted into triglycerides. What this means is that eating fruits will definitely work against ketosis and autophagy because it encourages the storage of liver glycogen. The content of glycogen in your liver is responsible for maintaining a balance between mTor and AMPK. The liver is more like a central hub for nutrients and metabolism. Eating fruits with fats and proteins that are regulated can help the body to remain a catabolic state of breaking down molecules even though there's a very slim chance of autophagy. While eating fruit is not bad, you need to restrict the amount of fruit you're eating if you have to maintain autophagy.

Chapter 6: Intermittent Fasting Protocols

One of the things that set intermittent fasting apart from other weight loss programs is the fact that there are many approaches to it. There are many choices you can make about the time or schedule you can follow that fits into your lifestyle. So whether you want to fast for a few hours a day or a couple of days a week, the choice is yours. Ultimately, there's no best way to do intermittent fasting because the underlying premise of how it works is the same, and every method has its own advantages and drawbacks. Here is some insight into the seven most popular intermittent fasting methods:

The 16/8 Method (Leangains)

This is the most popular form of intermittent fasting that has its beginnings linked to Martin Berkhan, a Swedish bodybuilder and nutritionist. When followed in its true form, this method will see you maximize your muscle while cutting fat. According to Berkhan's explanation, the premise behind this method is simple; you have an eight-hour feeding window and a sixteen-hour fasting window that is complimented by some work out that focuses on strength training.

Interestingly, Berkhan doesn't advocate intermittent fasting for weight loss alone; rather, he uses it to build muscle as well as help his clients reach their goals of body recomposition. This method works and probably the most used and easy to adopt despite being complex. The beauty of using the Leangains intermittent fasting protocol is that it's not a one size fits all plan; hence, you can tweak it to suits your needs. The tweaking mostly applies to the meal timing as well as macronutrient breakdown. If this method works for you, you will not have trouble sticking to it as it will become part of your lifestyle.

Execution of the 16/8 Intermittent Fasting Protocol

In terms of execution, the 16/8 method requires you to not only put in work but also track everything. This can be a challenge in the beginning, especially if you're not used to journaling. However, this is the key to the best results. You can then decide on when you will fast and feed. According to Berkhan, the best time to begin your fasting window is the afternoon all through to half-past eight at night. This is because this window is socially compatible because it covers the period when you get to do a lot of social eating.

Moreover, the early hours of being in the fasted state are covered during sleep, which you've used to already. This means that you have eight hours of rest and another eight hours that you need to fast. You'll also have to forfeit breakfast, something many people believe that you're not supposed to skip because we're conditioned to believe that it's the most important meal of the day. You also need to determine when you'll work out. Berkhan offers three suggestions; you can work out when you wake up, after your first meal or after your second meal. Your workouts should be targeted at strength training. He further recommends that you limit yourself to three meals within the eight hours. If anything, it's almost impossible to have more than three meals within an 8-hour window. Make sure your post-workout meal is the largest, while more than sixty percent of your recommended daily caloric intake should be from this meal.

Most importantly, make sure that you maintain the caloric deficit or eat at maintenance. This means that you calculate your basal metabolic rate (BMR) to determine the number of calories it takes to maintain your body. When calculating your BMR, you'll need to indicate your activity level. Make sure you pick the level you're at and go a level lower unless you're sedentary. It's common to underestimate how active you are so this approximation is sensible. A deficit would mean five hundred calories less this number while maintenance would be this number of calories. This means that if you eat this number of calories, you'll maintain. If you're able to keep up with 16/8 and work out, you can be sure to recompose your body and replace fat with muscle. You don't have to worry if you have a lot of weight to lose because when you begin losing fat, you'll slim down because your muscle is denser than fat.

You also need to think about the food you will eat and in what proportions. You can use online calculators to estimate the size of the portion as well as calories in your meals to be sure that it meets the total number required. It's up to you to determine how much of the food you eat will comprise of protein and what proportion will be carbs. If you choose to incorporate the keto diet, make sure you're taking a higher proportion of fat than carbs. Don't worry about putting on fat because your insulin levels will be low because of fasting, thus burning fat. Carbs are important in making progress during your work out because they fuel your muscles. When you follow through all these, make sure you track your measurements and weight, particularly your waist. If you realize you're not losing weight or you're gaining weight, you need to reduce the intake by 500 calories before you can begin tracking again.

Make sure you consume sixty percent of your total calorie intake post work out. This is important since your body is well trained to convert food into muscle after work out. Make sure you're avoiding fasted training because it's not only taxing but also presents high chances of burnout. Thus, it may mean that you take supplements so that you end up with too many things to track. You're better off sticking to working out in between your meals. Besides, working out in the evening and ending your fast at 8 p.m. will make sure you're getting a good night sleep because your body is tired physically. In conclusion, the Leangains way of intermittent fasting is an excellent method that is adaptable.

Tips to Make 16/8 a Success

Following through the Leangains intermittent fasting protocol is not as easy as it may seem. In fact, it can be a challenge. However, you can post very good results by following the following tips:

- Make sure you include an adequate amount of proteins in your meals during the feeding window. Try not to compensate for low protein intake you may have had on one day.

- If you must consume carbs, let it be on the days when you work out so that you burn the excess glucose.

- You must work out with this program

- Focus on eating nutrient-dense meals as opposed to calorie bombs that have little nutritional value. Most importantly, don't consume any calories during the fasting window. You can only drink water, take tea or coffee that is not sweetened.

- Don't eat before you work out but make sure that you eat a nutrient-dense meal post-workout.

Overall, it's up to you whether you'll have an eight hour or six-hour feeding period. Although there's no restriction on the number of carbs you can consume in a day, you'll do well to cut on carbs to make this program more effective.

The Warrior Diet

This diet is the brainchild of Ori Hofmekler and is proof of just how the human body is resilient. If you follow this method to the later and with discipline, you'll have a different perspective of the amount of food you need and the frequency with which you need it for your body to function well. This method of fasting is a lot more stringent than Leangains. With the warrior diet, your feeding window is further shortened to 4 hours while the fasting window is lengthened by 4 hours to make it 20 hours. This leaves means that you're likely to have a single meal or one and a half at most. While it seems impractical, this diet is perhaps the most effective when you look at it from the point of view of getting results. The only disadvantage is that you have to stick to it to get those results, and this is a struggle for most people. It is not difficult to get started with this diet because the internet is awash with information on how to go about it. Owing to the rather harsh nature of this plan, it mostly attracts people who are considered to have a tough personality that can handle it. In fact, you'll hardly receive support or sympathy online if you happen to be struggling with adherence. Because of this, it's common practice, to begin with, this intermittent fasting protocol before switching to a friendlier plan. Remember, the real issue with the warrior diet is mostly psychological with the potential of damaging your relationship with food. For instance, some people end up binge eating soon after giving up on this plan.

Execution of the Warrior Diet Intermittent Fasting Protocol

The first step in the implementation of the warrior diet is calculating your BMR and determine the number of calories you'll be getting from protein, fat, and carbs. Begin with the protein and then decide on your carbs and finally the remainder of the calories. You also must decide when you'll work out, taking into account the duration of your fasting window. While it's recommended that you only get into a heavy workout in the feeding phase, this can be difficult logistically because the time you dedicate to the gym alone is nearly half of your feeding duration. Moreover, the size of your meals will be bigger, so you need to have adequate time to eat and allow for digestion to take place. On the other hand, if you opt to fast in the fasted state, it's unlikely that you'll attain the performance that meets the demands of strength training regardless of the supplements you'll ingest.

Let's take a closer look; your body needs nutrition after close to twenty hours of fasting. Thus, working out in a fasted state only increases this need so you'll wait longer. Yet working out after a single meal means your workout will end towards the end of your feeding window. To balance this out, you'll need to shorten the length of your workout to preserve your muscle mass while increasing your fitness. This makes a high-intensity interval training (HIIT) workout ideal because it pushes your heart rate up to 90% of its maximum ability for a short interval leaving you with a slightly longer resting interval. You can repeat this for about 15 to 20 minutes. The advantage of a HIIT is that you're at liberty to do any movement as long as you do it with high intensity. From cycling, sprinting, jump rop0e, pushups, and squats, the options are endless. Make sure you're keeping the weight you're lifting so that you don't invite an injury. As you get used to it, you can reduce the rest interval to the point where its half of the size of the work out interval. The only challenge is that you'll develop the strength to a certain level then taper off. Although you will not hit a fat loss plateau during fasting, you will also not build muscle past a certain point. So, you can do HIIT four times and at least one day of fasted strength training even though you'll need supplements. If you think you have great willpower, keep in mind that the only easiest routine you can implement is one that requires the least change.

The Eat Stop Eat Method (5:2)

Brad Pilon, a bodybuilder, created this intermittent fasting routine. It pretty much imitates the ancient way of fasting. In fact, this method has many similarities with the ancient way of fasting in many ways. There aren't too many resources on the internet about this intermittent fasting protocol. In fact, most of the content you'll find online are affiliate marketer reviews.

Nonetheless, this method is very effective when you're getting into intermittent fasting because it's straight forward. That is; you eat regularly for five days and fast for the remaining two days. This means you have two blocks of a 24 hour fast during which you consume zero calories making it difficult to implement in reality because you can drink water, tea, and coffee.

The common fear with this method of intermittent fasting is that you might end up binge eating once you come to the end of your fasting window. Even then, studies have shown that the excess calories you consume post fasting do not qualify to warrant it being referred to as binge eating. However, it's important to make sure that you spread out your fasting days so that there's a realistic gap between them.

Execution of the 5:2 Intermittent Fasting Protocol

This method is often a good starting point to your intermittent fasting journey because the rules that govern it are more favorable. The requirements are also minimal. For instance, while Brad Pilon advocates for exercises, you don't have to go for HIIT or strength training. All you need to do is break a sweat and move. Hence this method is usually attractive to beginners. Although it's a good idea to know your maintenance calories, it's not a strict requirement because the days when you're fasting will mostly take care of all the excess calories you consume on feeding days. As such, this method motivates beginners to know that they can pull through without being under pressure. However, the result of this is that the weight loss will not be rapid, as is the case with Leangains and the warrior methods of intermittent fasting. Even then, you must be keen on following the guidelines so that you see the results.

Interestingly, there's a high tendency of flouting the guidelines of this method, especially by beginners than the guidelines of the warrior diet. This is because of a lack of understanding of how nutrition works. For this reason, this intermittent fasting method is not usually the best out there despite its efficacy.

Alternate Day Fast (36/12 Hour Fast)

This method of intermittent fasting promotes fasting for an extended period. This program was developed by a doctor/nutritionist Dr. James B. Johnson. As the name suggests, this plan recommends a feeding window of 12 hours, followed by 36 hours of fasting. This means that you can have all your three main meals in a day. Despite the extension in the fasting hours, this plan is doable. Even then, make sure that you eat nutrient-dense foods in the 12 hour feasting period. Your intake of proteins and healthy fats should be higher compared to your consumption of carbs. This program doesn't mention anything about working out, perhaps because of the extended hours of fasting. However, you can be sure to have better results with fasting. This method is also not as strict as it allows you to eat just about everything as long as it's healthy. Ultimately, eating nutrient-dense food is recommended as opposed to calorie-dense food.

Execution of the 36/12 Intermittent Fasting Protocol

The success of the alternate-day intermittent fasting method begins with establishing your fasting and feeding windows. That is, establish your feeding phase of 12 hours during the day. This means that you can have your first meal at 7 a.m. and the last at 7 p.m. on Monday and repeat this schedule 4 times a week. That is Monday, Wednesday, Friday and Sunday. You also need to define your fasting hours. These will typically begin after your last meal. In this case, it will be 7 p.m. all the way to Wednesday morning when you have your next feeding window.

The alternate-day intermittent fasting has worked for many people. This method will not only contribute to weight loss but also have a positive effect on overall health. Those who've tried this program have had up to 8 percent weight loss in a period of 8 weeks. Other benefits realized include better cellular energy production and improved insulin resistance. This intermittent fasting protocol is also deemed as the right program if you're keen on inducing autophagy or ease arthritis. Generally, 36 hours of fasting can be too radical for women. Thus, it's recommended that you have a slight intake of calories. If you opt to go this way, you need to limit your calorie intake to 20% of your normal calorie intake in the first two weeks and increase it to 35% afterward. From this perspective, feeding days are referred to as up days while the fasting days are down days. Some of the foods you can consume during the down days include smoothies and fruits. You must focus on eating healthy food during the eating window. Combing this program with exercise such as strength training will enhance fat burning hence better results.

Advantages of Alternate Day Fasting

The alternate-day fasting method offers plenty of advantages that include the following:

- Improved metabolism and extended lifespan.
- It helps in improving conditions like asthma.
- It's a doctor's idea; hence, it can be trusted to be good for your health.
- You don't have the challenge of deprivation since you can eat anything during your feeding window.
- This method is easy to follow over a long time.
- It's devoid of stringent rules in terms of food even though it recommends health eating.

Disadvantages of Alternate Day Fasting

Alternate day fasting presents a number of disadvantages that include:

- It's not recommended for people who have a history of eating disorders like anorexia.
- This intermittent fasting method doesn't discuss the importance of exercising or working out, which has a role in fat burning.
- When you practice this method, you have a high risk of experiencing dizziness, fatigue, and hunger, especially in the

first few days.

Crescendo Fasting

The female body is highly sensitive to signals of starvation compared to the male body. Because of this, fasting for long durations can trigger hormonal imbalances resulting in fatigue, hunger pangs, weight gain, and mood swings. Of all the intermittent fasting methods, crescendo fasting is most suited for women because it's less demanding on their bodies. This method does not require you to fast daily but 2 to 3 non-consecutive days for between 12 to 16 hours weekly. This means that you can maintain your regular feeding schedule on the days when you're not fasting. With this intermittent fasting protocol, you will be fasting three times weekly. You should avoid engaging in heavy workouts on the days when you're fasting and instead consider yoga or cardio. You can do intense exercise like HIIT and strength training on the days when you're fasting.

Advantages of Crescendo Fasting

Crescendo fasting presents a number of advantages that include the following:

-This intermittent fasting plan is gentle on the female body; thus, it preserves the hormonal balance that is crucial in a woman's life.

-Crescendo fasting prepares you for the other complicated intermittent fasting methods like alternate day fasting, eat stop eat, and warrior method mentally and physically.

-Crescendo fasting is an excellent method of burning fat pockets and slimming down in a manner that is not so difficult.

Disadvantages of the Crescendo Fasting

-When practicing crescendo fasting, you're likely to experience an irregular menstrual cycle. If this happens, please stop immediately.

-Crescendo fasting is also not good when you have eating disorders.

The 12/12 Intermittent Fasting Method

This is by far the easiest intermittent fasting protocol because it's simple. It's particularly great when you're beginning intermittent fasting. As the name suggests, you'll have a 12-hour fasting window followed by another 12-hour eating window. This is pretty easy to cope with because most of the fasting window is covered while you're sleeping. As such, you rarely feel hungry. The toughest part is that you have to limit your meal times to 3 times a day. However, you can counter this by making equal feeding intervals so that you're able to comfortably pass from one meal to another without having to eat snacks. This doesn't dispute the health benefits that come with intermittent fasting. Being on a 12 hour fast will give your system a great rest. Moreover, your insulin resistance will go down, thus activating the weight loss process.

It's not unusual to experience uneasiness, a slight headache, or nausea at the onset of your fasting. However, there's no cause for alarm because this is just a reaction to the withdrawal of sugar that is contrary to your regular habit of frequent snacking and glucose supply it gets. The body will try to adjust to this change, but you can also take unsweetened fresh lime, water, coffee, and black tea. These beverages are non-caloric in nature; hence, you can consume them without worrying about calories. Even then, you should not overindulge in caffeine as it can make you uneasy. You can follow through this intermittent fasting protocol for at least a fortnight before switching to another intermittent fasting protocol.

Tips to Maintain the Intermittent Fasting Lifestyle

Sticking to an intermittent fasting program can be quite a challenge. Here are some of the tips that will help you to stay on the track and maximize the benefits of this eating pattern:

Avoid obsessing over food. When you embark on intermittent fasting, you need to plan your day so that you're busy enough to distract you from thinking about food. This may be anything from catching up on some movie or doing some paperwork.

Stay hydrated. Drinking plenty of water and other calories free drinks like herbal teas throughout the day is a great way of keeping you full and strong so that you don't end up feeling too weak and hungry to give in to cravings.

Resting and relaxing. Although your body will tap into your fat stores for energy when you're fasting, it's advisable that you avoid strenuous activities. You can, however, consider light exercises like yoga.

Eat high volume foods. Make sure you're eating low calorie but filling foods during your feeding window, especially fruits that have a high percentage of water like melon and grapes as well as vegetables.

Make every calorie count. If your choice of an intermittent fasting plan allows you to sneak in a few calories, go for nutrient-dense foods that are rich in fiber, protein, and healthy fats. These include lentils, beans, fish, eggs, avocado, and nuts.

Choose nutrient-dense foods during your feeding window. Eating foods that are rich in minerals, vitamins, fiber, and other nutrients. This helps in keeping your sugar levels steady while preventing nutrient deficiencies. A balanced diet will also contribute to good overall health and weight loss.

Increase the taste without calories. You can season your meals generously with herbs, vinegar, spices, and garlic. These are full of flavor yet high in calories hence can help in suppressing the feeling of hunger.

Chapter 7: Transitioning Into Intermittent Fasting

If you're used to the pattern of eating where you eat after every 2-3 hours, transitioning into intermittent fasting can be a challenge. However, when you have the right approach, easing into intermittent fasting shouldn't be a problem. Here's how to ease into with intermittent fasting:

Get your doctor's nod. Before you begin the intermittent fasting lifestyle, you need to get a nod from your doctor. This is good even if you don't have a prevailing medical condition. Your doctor will advise you if you have any issues of concern that could pose a challenge to your health. This may including getting blood work done in addition to an all-round checkup.

Have a goal. Intermittent fasting presents so many benefits. However, it would be unrealistic to have them all as your goal for adopting this lifestyle. Therefore, you'll do well to have a goal that will be your point of reference during the period you'll be doing intermittent fasting. This may be weight loss, improving your metabolic health, or even improving your overall health. Having an ultimate goal helps you to determine an intermittent fasting method that will enable you to meet this goal. It also helps you to stay on course even when faced with cravings and are on the verge of giving up.

Identify a suitable intermittent fasting method. Not all the intermittent fasting methods are suitable for everyone, especially in terms of physiology. Even better, not all methods can help you achieve your specific goal of fasting. Therefore, take time to understand the different intermittent fasting methods before selecting a plan that suits your preferences. You also need to go for a plan that you can easily stick to without struggling too much. While intermittent fasting doesn't give restrictions on what foods you should eat and which ones you should avoid, you'll do well to focus on healthy high fiber whole foods and vegetables during your fasting window.

Know your caloric needs. One of the mistakes that many people make is jumping into the intermittent fasting lifestyle without knowing their daily caloric needs. If you're particularly interested in losing weight, you need to create a calorie deficit by consuming fewer calories than you're using. On the other hand, if you want to gain weight in the process, then you must consume more calories than your body can use. You can use the free online calorie calculators to be able to determine your daily calorie needs. Most importantly, your focus should be on nutrient-dense foods. This doesn't mean that you completely abandon junk; rather, you can eat it in moderation.

Create a meal plan. Depending on your goal of intermittent fasting, creating a meal plan will help you to stay focused and avoid eating foods that you had not intended but can interfere with your plan. This is not to say that you make your meal plan restrictive; instead, a meal plan will ensure you include all the nutrients you need now that you have less feeding times in a day.

Transition slowly. It's absolutely normal to be ambitious when getting into intermittent fasting. However, you'll do well not to make immediate changes to your eating schedule because this will only send your body into shock and exacerbate the side effects of withdrawing food. As such, you need to get into it gradually. This means that you begin by fasting for a few hours, gradually increasing them to the time when you can fast for 16 hours. While at it, you can also cut down on your consumption of junk food, especially if you're practicing intermittent fasting to lose weight. Starting with the most extreme intermittent fasting method is akin to setting yourself up to fail.

Review your diet. Although intermittent fasting continues to be advocated for because of benefits like leniency and flexibility that lets you eat just about anything, your efforts will not pay off if you fill your plate with junk food during your feeding window. This means that as part of your transition into this lifestyle, you must also take your diet into consideration. Focus on filling your plate with healthy food options like enough protein, healthy fats as well as complex carbohydrates while limiting highly processed carbs. This will no doubt make your transition smooth and easier because you'll feel full for longer when you fuel properly during your feasting window. Consequently, you're unlikely to struggle with some of the side effects of intermittent fasting that include feeling dizzy, hungry, and tired.

Avoid the temptation to overeat. After staying for long hours without eating, you'll naturally have the temptation to overeat once your eating window begins. You must be careful not to eat too much because this can result in a feeling of sickness, bloating, and cause weight gain. This is why counting your calories and having a meal plan come in handy because you can moderate what you're eating while avoiding excesses.

Track your progress. Unless you're beginning with the more complex intermittent fasting methods with extended hours of fasting, then don't set your expectations of weight loss too high in the first few weeks. Therefore, you'll do well to keep a journal by writing down your progress as well as how you feel physically and emotionally. You also need to take photos before you start and as you by while also tracking your weight. This helps you to stay on track and stay motivated so that you don't give up.

Chapter 8: Mistakes You Should Avoid During Intermittent Fasting

There's no doubt that intermittent fasting comes with many benefits that enhance your overall wellbeing. It's important to keep in mind that you'll not realize these benefits overnight. You need to be patient and disciplined while avoiding mistakes that are likely to make your transition into intermittent fasting difficult. Here are some common mistakes people make when transitioning to the intermittent fasting lifestyle and how you can fix them:

Transitioning to intermittent fasting too fast. If you haven't been fasting, then chances are that you're used to eating at least every 3-4 hours. When you suddenly decide to extend this window to 8 hours or more, you'll end up feeling hungry, weak, and discouraged during the entire period of fasting. Eventually, you'll have to quit because you can no longer cope with the effects of the fast. You need to begin the transition gradually by increasing the hours of your fast after every two days or so. Do this until you're able to fast for 12 hours or until you reach your goal. This way, your body is able to adjust to the new changes smoothly without interfering with your lifestyle. Remember, it'll take a while before you stop feeling hungry whenever you're fasting.

Overeating during your feasting window. This is a trap that most people fall into when they first practice intermittent fasting. When you've chosen an intermittent fasting protocol that leaves you hungry for so many hours, you'll most likely go overboard when it's time to eat. This is because you're emotionally starved more than you actually feel hungry. Sometimes you just could be feeling ravenous, or you're simply justifying it by the thought that after all, you're making up for the lost calories. Therefore, you need to make sure that you carry on with your life as usual so that you are not preoccupied with your next meal during the fasting window as to feel hungry unnecessarily. This will backfire if your main goal of practicing intermittent fasting is weight loss, but you are overeating during your feasting window. You can avoid this pitfall by making sure you prepare a healthy meal and have it ready by the time your fasting window ends. Be sure to include whole ingredients and healthy carbs such as whole grains, plenty of vegetables as well as lean protein.

Choosing the wrong plan for your lifestyle. Let's face it; we all have a different lifestyle with different commitments. However, you may end up choosing a plan that doesn't fit into your lifestyle because of too much ambition to achieve the results you desire quickly. By selecting an intermittent plan that doesn't align with your lifestyle, you're just setting yourself up for failure and making a bad situation worse. Don't go for a plan that will cramp your life. For instance, if you're a night owl, then you should consider a plan that lets you fast during the day when you're less active as opposed to starting your fast at 6 p.m. On the other hand, if you're into gym workouts and you can't sacrifice your morning workout or your daily spin, then you need to consider a plan that doesn't restrict calories severely for a few days in the week.

Not eating enough during the eating window. While most people will struggle with eating too much when it's time to eat, others eat too little. Although you want to assume that by eating too little, you'll lose more weight, the reverse is true. You might actually end up gaining weight. When you're not eating enough, you jeopardize your chances of making progress; you'll fail. Eating too little will cannibalize your muscle mass, resulting in a slowed-down metabolism. The lack of metabolic muscle mass will sabotage your ability to retain fat in the future. This is one of the challenges that intermittent fasting presents because you're eating according to some rules as opposed to following your body's innate cues. As a result, you're unable to know your actual needs. If you're not sure about how much is too much or too little, then you can speak to a registered dietician to get help in assessing your nutritional needs and how best to meet them safely.

Not drinking the right liquids. When you're fasting, you're at liberty to drink fluids. In fact, it's important to make sure you're well hydrated. The most advocated for liquids during fasting are water, tea, and black coffee that are unsweetened. You can add a splash of milk in your coffee if you can't stand black coffee. However, you need to understand the importance of keeping off coconut oil and butter. Other liquids that you must keep away from include protein filled liquids like bone broth since they have the potential of halting autophagy from taking place. Remember, one of the aims of intermittent fasting is promoting autophagy; the cellular process responsible for breaking down and recycling damaged molecules.

Similarly, you've got to give up diet sodas as well as other sweetened drinks even if they're calorie-free. Experts have found that zero-calorie sweeteners often have a negative effect on the level of insulin, thereby stimulating appetite so that you constantly want to eat. You can use an app to track your hydration and be accountable.

Being sedentary. If you're used to having a pre-workout snack before hitting the gym, then the idea of exercising while fasting may appear to be foreign. As such, you may end up retreating to being sedentary. What most people often forget is that you have enough energy stored in your body in the form of body fat that you used in the absence of food. This means that it's safe to exercise when fasting. Even then, just like it is with any exercise or diet plan always make sure you seek the advice of your doctor before you incorporate exercise into your intermittent fasting lifestyle. You need to keep up with your usual workout plan or reduce the intensity of your workout sessions. You can settle for less intensive exercise plans, like walking. You can also schedule your intermittent fasting plan so that your exercise time falls within the fasting window. Most importantly, make sure you're eating protein-rich foods that will help to build muscle fast.

Not drinking enough liquids. Although your intermittent fasting plan requires you to refrain from eating food during the fasting period, you can take fluids. In fact, it's recommended that you drink up as much water to stay hydrated. So you need to make sure that you always have water nearby because you're missing hydration from foods like vegetables and fruits. Failure to hydrate well can result in muscle cramps and headaches as well as exacerbate hunger pangs. So you should keep sipping during your fast.

Eating unhealthy foods during the eating window. It's not automatic that you will lose weight because you're doing intermittent fasting. Therefore, you should not make intermittent fasting an excuse to make unhealthy food choices. Although intermittent fasting focuses on when you eat but seems to be silent on the nutritional quality of the food you eat, it's advisable that you stick to healthy food choices. In fact, it's important to pay attention to the nutritional value of the food you're eating to make sure that you're not nutrient deficient. Your nutritional needs don't change with fasting. This means that by consuming processed foods instead of whole foods, you're compromising a well-balanced diet. As a result, intermittent fasting will not help you in reaching your goal of losing weight and leading a healthy lifestyle. Tracking the food you eat, and when you eat, it will make a huge difference in your intermittent fasting journey.

Failure to fast properly during the fasting period. When you are fasting, you need to consume zero or close to zero calories. Even then, you could accidentally slip them in, and when this happens, it breaks your fast, thus slowing down your efforts. Take the example of a cup of tea or coffee; you can have it as long as it doesn't have calories. Generally, a cup of tea shouldn't break you fast if it doesn't exceed 50 calories. Therefore, if you're having black coffee, you can add a dash of milk. This means that if you prefer that caramel latte to satisfy your sweet tooth, then you could be breaking your fast.

Attempting to do many things at once. If you've been trying to lose weight for some time, then the allure of the benefits of intermittent fasting can be so tempting that you find yourself attempting to do just about everything. Unfortunately, this is often counterproductive because you just might end up putting on weight instead. Refrain from the desire of doing everything. For instance, don't start intermittent fasting at the same time you're starting a new training program or a new diet. Always focus on making gradual progress. For instance, if you'd like to combine both training and intermittent fasting, then begin by extending your hours or fasting gradually until you get to a point where you're comfortable. You can start with one day of training and advance to more days over time. Otherwise combining so many changes at once can result in problems because you'll experience physical stress.

Obsessing over timings and eating windows. When you begin intermittent fasting, you might be overwhelmed and feel nervous. This is because you don't know if you'll have the ability to pull through or you'll post poor results just like it is with other diets. As a result of this, you might end up obsessing over intermittent fasting and the anticipated results. This is not good because when you fast and go about your business, as usual, you give your body an opportunity to adjust to the program accordingly. That is, it can tell when you'll experience real hunger and when you actually get to eat. On the contrary, when you think too much about your fast and how long it is before you get to eat, your body doesn't learn the signals.

Doing an intense workout during your fast. While it is recommended that you don't lead a sedentary lifestyle when you're practicing intermittent fasting, you shouldn't engage in an intense workout. In fact, you should avoid doing anything that is too taxing on an empty stomach such as high-intensity workout. It's dangerous to engage in an intense workout when you don't have fuel in your system. Therefore, make sure you schedule your workouts within your eating window or simply settle for a low-intensity workout when you're fasting.

Giving up too soon. While it may seem easy compared to following a diet, intermittent fasting is not a walk in the park because you'll have to go on with your daily activities on fewer calories than usual. This means going without food for longer hours than usual. In the beginning, you're bound to experience challenges regardless of the intermittent fasting protocol you choose. You may experience exhaustion, irritability, or even general body weakness. When this happens, most people throw in the towel instead of holding on and letting their bodies adjust to the new pattern of eating.

Forcing intermittent fasting to work for you. Although it's true that intermittent fasting will produce certain results like weight loss and longevity, you must remember that it doesn't work for all. Therefore, if you have tried it, but it only makes you feel miserable, then you can take time to re-evaluate if it's the best approach you can use to achieve your goals. Remember, that while some bodies can handle starvation pretty well just like our ancestors, others can't.

Being unreasonably strict. It's likely that you're too strict when you begin intermittent fasting in that you can't even think of ending your fat a little earlier. You need to be more realistic as opposed to just following through the program because there are times you may have to break your fast earlier than usual, which is fine. Keep in mind that no one is perfect; thus, when you loosen up, you'll take off pressure off yourself. This will give you more chances of succeeding with the program because you'll be less stressed; hence, you can stick with the program for long.

Chapter 9: Common Myths about Intermittent Fasting

There's no question about the fact that intermittent fasting has attracted a huge following owing to the benefits associated with it. However, there are several unfounded misconceptions and myths surrounding this pattern of eating. These myths provide wring information and are sometimes the reason many people shy away from trying intermittent fasting either for weight loss or a wholesome lifestyle. This chapter debunks some of the common unfounded claims about intermittent fasting to help you make the most of this practice. Here are some of the common myths about intermittent fasting:

Intermittent fasting makes you binge eat. This claim is far from the truth because it classifies intermittent fasting under eating disorders while classifying people who eat every two hours as being normal. The thing that intermittent fasting pays attention to is whether you're meeting your daily macronutrient and calorie goals. For some people, this may mean eating a large meal. This doesn't necessarily mean you're leaning towards binge eating.

Moreover, when you fast you tap into a multitude of benefits, thus to say that by practicing intermittent fasting, you're likely to end up binge eating is a misrepresentation. Realistically speaking, it would be unfair to think that you just need to eat a few nuts or raisins when you're doing intermittent fasting and call it a day because then you'll not meet your daily caloric needs. In a nutshell, when you're fasting, you'll have to pack more nutrients per meal hence eating a large meal portion isn't equivalent to binge eating. If anything, binge eating means eating in an uncontrollably gluttonous way.

Intermittent fasting makes you lose muscle. The idea that your body requires a constant supply of amino acids to maintain, repair, or build muscle tissue; hence, fasting will result in the breakdown of muscle tissues for energy is untrue. In reality, the fact that you're fasting doesn't mean that your body is in a catabolic mode. What is often overlooked by proponents of this idea is that it's possible to have a large bolus of slow-digesting proteins from your last meal releasing amino acids by the time you're breaking your fast. In fact, it's not uncommon to have a complete meal consisting of more than 100 grams of slow-digesting proteins that will carry you through the next eating window. However, don't lose sight of the fact that when you fast for extended periods, you'll most certainly lose a bit of muscle because your liver glycogen and amino acids are likely to be depleted. Even then, this is unlikely to occur if you're fasting for 16-20 hours because you generally eat a large balanced meal at every feasting window.

Intermittent fasting is only applicable to limited populations. This is actually a laughable claim because intermittent fasting is more applicable to most people's lifestyles compared to the regular pattern of eating round the clock. Most people who opt to follow through the intermittent fasting lifestyle find it to be a huge relief from having to obsessively follow through the clock throughout the day just to make sure they're eating after every 2-3 hours. It's undeniable that most people's daily routines favor intermittent fasting because you don't always have the time to have full meals throughout the day. You're likely to be preoccupied with getting ready to go rather than getting something to eat in the morning contrary to the idea that has been advanced over the years that breakfast is the most important meal of the day. It's also worth noting that not many people prefer eating a large meal in the morning or even in the middle of busy work or school day. In essence, this means that at any one point so many people practice intermittent fasting, albeit, unknowingly. For most people, it's more convenient to go about the day without worrying about food. This doesn't mean that regular feeding isn't viable or applicable, rather it debunks the misconception that intermittent eating isn't pragmatic and doesn't apply to a wide population.

Intermittent fasting will decrease your training performance. If you're a training enthusiast, the thought of intermittent fasting will definitely be the last thing on your mind. In fact, for most people, the immediate reaction to the idea of switching to the intermittent fasting lifestyle is that the two don't go hand in hand since performance will be hindered when your body is nutrient deprived. Studies were done on athletes who were training while fasting during the Ramadhan revealed that intermittent fasting doesn't hinder aerobic and anaerobic performance. It's also worth noting that intermittent fasting doesn't advocate for abstinence from water or non-caloric drinks during the fasting window. Therefore, dehydration shouldn't be a concern. Should you realize that your performance isn't as great when you're fasting, it's most certainly because of a subjective or psychological issue. If you're also not adapted to training without eating, then you just might give up before you get used to training when fasting. This is because you'll feel weak, sluggish, and hungry. These signals usually dissipate with time even as your performance peaks again. Most importantly, keep in mind that you don't have to work out during your fasted state; you can actually schedule eating pattern so that you train after a pre-workout shake or meal.

Frequent Eating Boosts Metabolism. Cutting down on the number times or rescheduling your meal times to accommodate intermittent fasting isn't about restricting calories. It's deliberate about when you eat. While it's largely assumed that reducing your meal times will result in slow metabolism, the truth is waiting for a few hours before you can have your first meal doesn't affect your metabolic rate. Fasting for short-term periods of up to 72 hours will actually increase your body's resting metabolic rate because of the release of norepinephrine.

Intermittent fasting will put your body in starvation mode. Fasting is not the same as starvation because when you fast, you're only changing the times when you eat so that you give the body what it needs when it needs. Recent research has found that you have to refrain from eating for up to three who days before your body can begin lowering your resting metabolic rate. Starvation is as a result of the body using up all the stored body fat that is used as energy. As a result, you cannibalize your muscles and other vital organs for survival. This will not happen when you skip a meal or two. The human body has the capacity to withstand periods without food because fat is stored energy, while the muscle is the functional tissue. Therefore, when you don't eat food for a certain duration, your body will begin burning fat resulting in weight loss. However, when you prolong the fasting period unreasonably, then your body will begin breaking down muscle. Your muscles store glycogen and glucose from food in the liver and muscle for short-term energy, while fat is stored for long-term storage.

Women can't fast. It's largely assumed that the reason women can't fast is that they're more sensitive to signals of starvation compared to men. When your body senses that it's being starved then it ramps up production of hunger hormones ghrelin and leptin. This is what women mostly feel when they are experiencing insatiable hunger when you don't eat enough. It's actually the hormones that bring about this feeling. This is the female body's way of protecting a potential fetus even when you're not pregnant.

In most cases, a negative energy balance is to blame for hormonal changes in women as and not only how much food you're eating. Other factors that can lead to negative energy include poor nutrition, excessive exercise, too much stress, too little rest/recovery, illness, and chronic inflammation or infection. These stressors are enough to put your body into negative energy balance that eventually affects your hormones.

You can eat all you want during the feasting window. This is a major pitfall for people who have tried intermittent fasting unsuccessfully because it ends up being a struggle. When you refrain from eating for a couple of hours doesn't mean that you eat whatever you want during the feasting window. The whole idea of losing weight during intermittent fasting is a result of a caloric deficit. You'll definitely struggle losing weight is you're exceeding your maintenance calories. There's a specific number of calories that your body burns throughout the day to maintain your current weight depending on your weight, height, age, and body fat. This means that eating more than that number of calories within the feasting window will result in weight gain regardless of how long you spend fasting. Therefore, you need to refrain from eating excessively but instead focus on eating a balanced diet that includes lots of vegetables, fruits, and lots of fiber. Avoid processed foods as well as foods that have too many preservatives and instead stick to wholesome, nutritious, and fresh foods.

When you fast, you'll be hungry all the time. When you talk about intermittent fasting, the biggest worry most people have is having to feel hungry all the time. Generally, it's frightening to think that you can stay between 16-20 hours without food every day. Most people will worry about being hungry every time until they break the fast. Well, you'll be surprised to know that this isn't the case. The truth is that while you will initially feel tired, hungry, and sluggish, you soon get used to the intermittent fasting period by questioning why you're going through it. Soon, your body will adjust to the new lifestyle effectively making changes to the manner in which your body operates. Over time, intermittent fasting will become much easier. The best way to incorporate it into your lifestyle is by beginning with shorter fasting of 14 hours, gradually advancing to 16 hours and later 18 hours or more. While at it, make sure you're listening to your body so that you don't end up straining.

Intermittent fasting is like magic. When you think through the benefits of practicing the intermittent fasting way of life, it feels like magic because of the quick and often visible results. This is because when it comes to weight loss, it usually takes time before you can begin seeing results. Intermittent fasting is not magic. It's based on science as many studies have been done analyzing its cause and effects. That is, when your body expends more calories than you're consuming, your body will be calorie deficient hence resulting in weight loss. Intermittent fasting also causes a decrease in the level of insulin levels that is instrumental in facilitating the burning of fat.

You shouldn't ingest anything during the fasting window. It's widely believed that you shouldn't ingest anything when you're fasting, including water. Well, the truth is that it's a bad idea to cut out on your water consumption just because you're fasting. You need to take water even when you're practicing intermittent fasting. And that is not all. You can also take other beverages that don't contain any calories like unsweetened tea and coffee because they'll not stimulate insulin. Remember, the whole idea behind intermittent fasting is that you get more benefits when your body is in a low oxygen state for longer. So feel free to have a cup of coffee. You can also consider ghee or butter because they have healthy fats that put your body in ketosis, thereby shifting your body's primary fuel from glucose to ketones.

Alternate day fasting is the best kind of fasting. There are various forms of intermittent fasting. For instance, with alternate-day fasting, you restrict your consumption of calories to less than 500 per day, all of which you consume in one meal. On the other hand, with the 5:2 intermittent fasting protocol, you will eat normally for five days and restrict your calories severely for two days. With the 16/8 intermittent fasting protocol, your fasting window lasts for 16 hours with the remaining 8 being your eating window. The best kind of fasting is not determined by the number of hours you're fasting, but how long you can fast and the benefits, you're seeking to achieve. For instance, if your goal is to achieve autophagy, then you'll definitely have to consider an intermittent fasting protocol that requires you to fast for extended periods.

You'll lose weight no matter what. Contrary to the belief that intermittent fasting does not always result in weight loss. This is a misconception because no matter how long you fast if you're still stuck on throwing down pizza, candy, or even burgers, then you shouldn't expect a difference in terms of weight loss. The reason there's an emphasis that intermittent fasting is a lifestyle is that it works hand in hand with a healthy diet. As such, don't expect to treat your fasting period like a cheat day and expect results.

Having frequent meal times will help reduce hunger. Most of the people who prefer to eat and snack frequently believe that it's a great way of preventing hunger so that you don't end up eating too much food. Several studies have looked into this, and the evidence is interesting. Some studies suggest that having frequent meals will reduce hunger while other studies found that there are not effects. Yet other studies also showed that eating frequently increased hunger levels. Ultimately, this depends on an individual — different strokes for different folks.

Skipping breakfast will make you fat. It's a common notion that breakfast is the most important meal of the day. As such, when you skip breakfast, you're likely to experience excessive hunger, cravings, and eventually gain weight. While a number of studies have found a link between skipping breakfast and obesity, this can be explained by the fact that a breakfast skipper is usually less health-conscious. A study done on 283 obese and overweight adults to determine the effect of skipping or eating breakfast found that there's no difference whether you eat or don't eat breakfast.

Eating many smaller meals will help lose weight. Eating many smaller meals does not boost metabolism/the calories that you burn.

Furthermore, they also don't help in reducing hunger/the amount of calories you consume. Therefore, if eating frequently doesn't have an effect on the energy balance equation, it shouldn't have an effect on weight loss. However, if eating more frequently will make it easier for you to eat fewer calories, it may be effective for you.

Your brain needs a constant supply of glucose. Some people believe that not eating carbs for a few hours will affect how your brain functions. This is based on the perception that the brain only uses glucose as fuel. Even then, they overlook the fact that your body can produce glucose whenever it needs through gluconeogenesis. In most cases, this is not needed because your body has glycogen stored in the liver for use when the brain needs it.

Conclusion

Thank you for making it through *Intermittent Fasting for Women*. I hope this book was informative, and you're now well equipped with the right information to take on intermittent fasting. Just because you've read this book doesn't mean you've mastered the entire intermittent fasting benefits. You actually need to put the information into practice in order to realize the results.

The next step is to stop reading and begin working out a plan of how to slowly and gradually getting into the intermittent fasting lifestyle without struggling. You can begin by analyzing your lifestyle and relate to the different intermittent fasting methods before creating a schedule you can follow. Remember, intermittent fasting should fit into your lifestyle and not the other way round. So you don't have to worry about making significant changes to accommodate the program. Remember, you can always try out a different intermittent fasting protocol if you feel the protocol you had initially selected doesn't suite you. Don't be too hard on yourself by having unrealistic expectations. The change doesn't happen overnight.

Keep in mind that exercise and training for strength are important in helping to create compounding gains and building muscle.

However, you don't have to complicate your workouts. Keep it simple. It's often easy to get derailed so you can keep on making reference to the many nuggets I have shared in this book to help you stay on track. I hope this book has shaped your perspective on intermittent fasting and that you're ready to get into it.

The Autophagy Diet

Remove Toxicity and Provide Energy to Obtain A Rapid Weight Loss and Anti-Aging Process Through Ketogenic Diet, Intermittent Fasting and Extended Water

By Agatha Franklin

Chapter 1: What is Autophagy?

Autophagy is a natural process that occurs in our body at a cellular level. It involves breaking down old, damaged cells and reusing them for fuel. Proteins and other materials contained in the destroyed cell matter are used to form new, stronger, and healthier cells. This is a fascinating event because it literally cleans up cell waste that would otherwise remain stored in our body. In simple terms, autophagy rejuvenates our body and provides many benefits as a result. Although autophagy has become a buzzword and an interesting topic of discussion among diet experts and professionals, it is far from being a new concept. The autophagy process begins at a point when our body requires fuel for building and repairing new cells and tissues. On a cellular scale, we use the nutrients and energy from the food we consume, usually in the form of glucose. When we consume a diet low in carbs, such as the ketogenic diet, we use up the glucose quickly, which is converted from the carbohydrates and switch to burning fat stores. Once we use all that we have, our body will continue to search for materials to break down and use. This is when autophagy takes effect: our body will identify old, damaged cellular waste and use it for energy.

In ancient societies, our ancestors benefitted from autophagy during long periods of fasting and eating whole foods low in carbohydrates and sugars, such as a wild game, berries and leafy greens, all of which could be hunted and gathered. Processed foods were not available, and our ancestors were more physically active, as this was the only means to obtain food. Periods of fasting would occur in between meals, as food could not be adequately stored as today, in refrigerators and freezers. Just over a century ago, people consumed more wholesome foods, as a ready-made, packaged meals only became popular once life became busier in the 1950s, leaving less time to prepare and enjoy foods in their natural state.

Thousands of years ago, when there was no food available for longer periods of time, people simply did not eat and had to search and seek out food sources available, in the form of foraging through forests and jungles to hunting. During these periods, people would naturally fast or abstain from food, which has benefits on its own and leads to the onset of autophagy, which is explained further in chapter ___. A clearer mind, and better focus and clarity, were considered among the benefits of fasting, as the food was a distraction. Fasting was also practiced in ancient times for other reasons as well, including for religious practices and spiritual reasons. During food shortage, or in between hunting and harvesting, fasting was a regular occurrence and circumstantial. Fasting can last from several hours during a 24-hour period to several days. It is currently practiced by many people in the form of intermittent fasting, which refers to extended periods of time between meals, though not necessarily for more than a day at a time.

The Autophagy Process

The basic science of how autophagy works to "clean" our bodies and rejuvenate cells. The word autophagy literally translates as "self-eating" or self-consuming. It is our body's way of developing a recycling program, making our bodies more efficient at identifying faulty or broken parts, including cancerous cells, and other materials that can cause or contribute to harm, such as obesity and chronic metabolic issues. The science behind autophagy is fascinating, and research is ongoing to determine the risks and benefits of its powerful effects. Also known as autophagocytosis, this occurs when proteins inside of the double-membrane vesicle inside cells, which are extracted and moved into the lysosome. Lysosomes are surrounded by a membrane, and also contain hydrolytic enzymes that work together to break down proteins, nucleic acids and other materials found in cells that can be recycled and reused in the building of new cells and tissues. Studies conducted in laboratories indicate that a significant reduction in caloric intake, and more specifically, fasting, will trigger this process. The results of this research indicate a decline in certain conditions in rats and mice, such as weight loss, increased longevity, and metabolism occurred after just twenty-four hours of fasting. At this time, high levels of autophagosomes were found in their bodies, indicating a state of autophagy.

During the autophagy process, two main hormones become involved: glucagon and insulin. As insulin levels rise, the level of glucagon decreases, and the same occurs in reverse: when glucagon increases, insulin falls. When glucagon rises, it stimulates the production of autophagosomes, and autophagy begins. The approximate time frame for inducing this process is a fast of approximately fifteen hours. This gives your body enough time to reduce insulin, though a longer fast means better results, which is usually closer to a full twenty-four hours. The role diet plays in our daily lives and how we schedule our meals has a significant impact on how we can benefit from autophagy and determining when it will work best to maximize its potential.

Chapter 2: How Does Autophagy Play a Role in Diet?

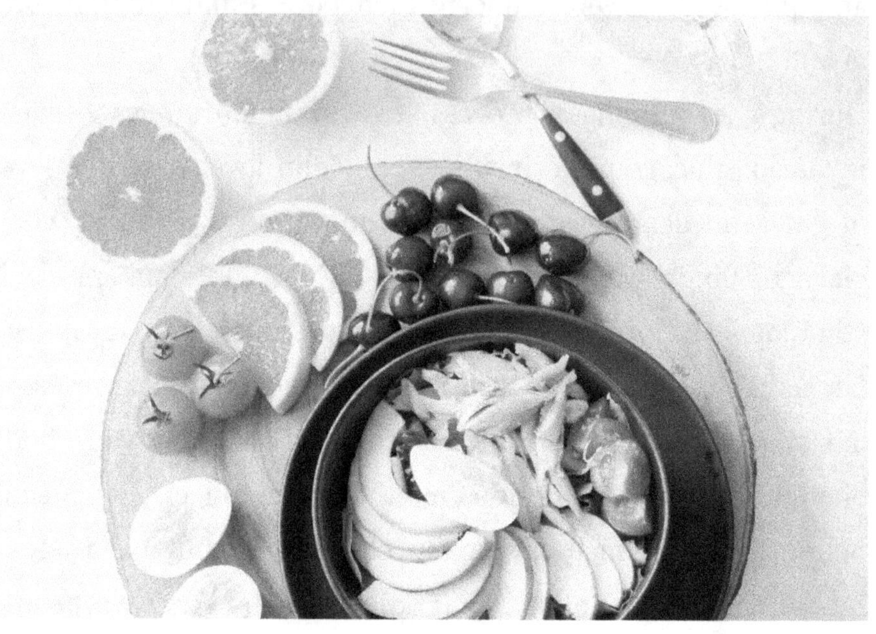

Autophagy plays a major role in our diet in several ways: what we eat and when we eat. These two factors, the what and when determine how quickly we can shift into a state of autophagy, and during which time frame within that window of opportunity is the most efficient and beneficial to reap the rewards of this cellular clean up process. To begin this process, it's best to prepare and plan ahead carefully and avoid "jumping" into an all-or-nothing approach, such as a 24-hour fast without any preparation or prior fasting experience or eliminating all high carb foods overnight with little to no options for replacement. One of the most important factors of the autophagy diet, as with any diet that is expected to make significant results, is to plan, prepare, and take time to adjust in stages. For example, going from a standard way of eating, which often includes a lot of sugars and carbohydrates, to a low carb, whole food diet with periods of intermittent fasting is a major shift, and your body will react accordingly. For this reason, it's best to begin the change in the diet gradually at a level that works best for you and your body.

How to Begin an Autophagy Diet

Beginning the autophagy diet is more of a process than a meal plan. This includes implementing several new ways of approaching diet and food planning to achieve a state of autophagy, by reducing the body's reliance on carbohydrates as the main fuel source and moving towards becoming fat adapted. During this phase, on a cellular level, your body will benefit from periods of fasting, which can occur in smaller time frames on a daily basis, or for longer periods of a day or more. Once your body is burning fat for fuel, shifting into fasting will take you towards achieving autophagy, where your body has used up its fuel sources and begins to search for the old, damaged cellular matter to use as energy.

To begin the journey to autophagy, consider the plan in stages, by first implementing either an intermittent fasting schedule or a low carb diet, both of which will limit your carb and calorie intake. Once you become comfortable with either the fasting schedule or diet, you can implement both, alternating between regular eating of low carb (preferably ketogenic) foods and periods of fasting.

Chapter 3: Why Choose Autophagy? The Benefits and Risks of this Diet

Are there risks as well as benefits to this diet? Can autophagy cause problems along with the positive results? The effects of autophagy are phenomenal and fascinating for many people, though there are also side effects and risks associated with intermittent fasting, low carb eating combined to reach this state. It is also not always a good choice for some people while remaining a significant benefit to others, for the following reasons:

- If you have an eating disorder of already established bad eating habits, such as skipping meals frequently, for this reason, intermittent fasting is not a good choice. The difference between fasting in between meals and skipping them is the planned and calculated approach, which is used in the fasting process, whereas skipping meals with little or no planning can be harmful, particularly if you don't eat the right foods or very small amounts in between skipping them. For intermittent fasting to work effectively, and lead to autophagy, a good, healthy way of eating should be established before moving into a fasting state, so that your body has enough nutrients available.

- If you have type 1 diabetes, it's important to maintain consistent insulin levels, which may be a challenge during intermittent fasting and a ketogenic diet. If you have this condition and are seriously considering an autophagy diet plan, it's best to consult a doctor first. Alternatively, progressing to a state of autophagy through intermittent fasting and low carb foods can prevent type 2 diabetes and control its progression in cases where it has already started. The difference between type 1 and 2 diabetes: type 1 is when the body doesn't produce enough or any insulin at all, and type 2 can vary from maintaining high insulin to not enough. Type 1 diabetes must be carefully monitored medically and requires regular doses of insulin, whereas the type 2 condition can be controlled and treated through a healthy diet, which is how low carb eating and fasting can be beneficial

- Intermittent fasting is not advised for women who are pregnant or breastfeeding. It's also best to avoid while trying to conceive. Low carb and ketogenic diets are best postpartum, instead of during pregnancy or breastfeeding, as our bodies need the extra fuel for energy.

- Anyone under the age of 18 should avoid the goal of

autophagy altogether. As you grow and develop, it's vital not to limit caloric intake or carbohydrates, unless under the supervision of a doctor for medical reasons. It is a goal best suited for adults for the purpose of improving health and losing weight. For older adults, autophagy is an ideal option to slow down the aging process, the benefits of which are covered in this book.

Overall, autophagy is a process that shouldn't be considered lightly and may take a while to work towards. The steps that lead to autophagy, intermittent, and long-term fasting, as well as ketogenic or low carb dieting, can take a while to adjust to if they are new concepts. Each step is a journey in itself, to explore and try different approaches, until you feel comfortable enough to progress further, with the ultimate goal of reaching autophagy.

Chapter 4: The Different Ways to Approach an Autophagy Diet

There are several paths to achieve autophagy, all of which reduce the caloric intake of foods, thereby reducing insulin and increasing the body's ability to shift into ketosis, which leads to producing autophagosomes. There are individual factors to consider, including the level of physical activity, current eating habits, and diet. Aside from achieving autophagy, there are beneficial ways to eat and fast that can support an easier shift to cellular rejuvenation, and an overall improvement in how your body feels and functions.

Extended water fasts

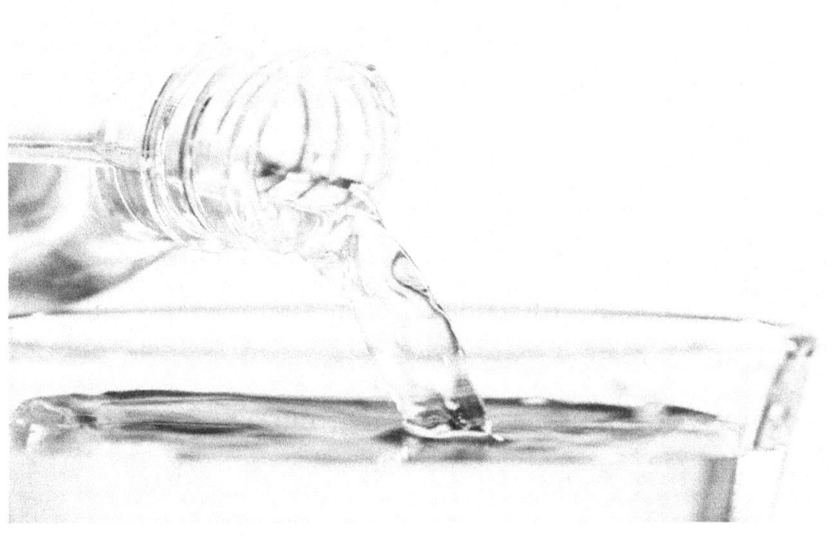

Fasting, more specifically, intermittent fasting, is one of the most effective methods of weight loss and encouraging autophagy. Water fasting essentially involves fasting for short or intermediate periods of time, while drinking lots of water to remain hydrated and flush toxins. This method of fasting restricts all foods and drinks, except water, for the duration of the fast. A water fast is beneficial for several reasons:

- It keeps hunger from developing. Water is often what we need when we experience hunger, which is one of the first signs of dehydration or thirst. Drinking water regularly, especially during a fast, reduces these false hunger pangs

- Even during short periods of water fasting, research indicates a reduction in blood pressure, cholesterol and heart disease, better metabolism, and weight loss.

- Improved concentration and energy. If your fast includes water that is filtered and re-mineralized (minerals are added back after removal with other elements), you'll continue to have the benefits of these nutrients while you abstain from food.

- Water fasting can be done easily from 24 hours for up to 3 days. It is recommended to begin with shorter periods of fasting, from 16 to 18 hours, prior to extending to one full day or more.

- Without the inclusion of carbohydrates during this fast, your body will use fat stores to burn for fuel and energy, which increases the potential for weight loss

Ketogenic Diet and the Basics of Ketosis

The ketogenic diet is a way of eating that centers around increasing the healthy fats while strictly reducing carbohydrates to less than (or up to) 20 grams per day. This diet was developed around the 1930s to treat many health conditions, such as seizures resulting from epilepsy, insulin regulation, and other diseases and conditions difficult to treat with conventional therapy. Reducing the carbohydrates significantly was the key to success for the treatments of these and many other conditions. Studies conducted in more recent years indicate numerous benefits, including fighting (and preventing) type 2 diabetes, brain, and cognitive function, preventing Alzheimer's and other related diseases. Weight loss and insulin regulation are two major results that have given the keto diet a significant amount of popularity recently, with many dieticians and medical professionals either supporting or criticizing the low carb way of eating.

Ketosis is a state that shifts your body's prime fuel source from carbohydrates and glucose to fats stored in the body. By reducing the number of carbs in your diet, the body will default to fat stores. During this process, the liver produces ketones, which indicates ketosis is in effect, and the body is fat adapted or in fat-burning mode. The ketones increase as the glucose falls, and the body has no other sources of energy. There are three types of ketones that result during this process:

- Acetoacetate (known as AcAc)
- 3beta-hydroxybutyrate (3HB)
- Acetone

The first two, AcAc and 3HB are the most abundant of the three, while acetone is produced during the body's expelling of ketones, and in trace amounts. The presence of ketones can be detected by test strips, which are often available at a pharmacy or drug store. Blood tests and testing the level of ketones in breath are two other methods, though test strips that detect ketones in urine are most popular and most accurate. While testing for ketones is not a requirement of the diet, it is often done to confirm the onset of ketosis and track its progress over a duration of time. The following scale is used to determine the level of ketosis, based on the production of ketones:

No ketosis	Trace amount	More than a trace, close to a small amount	Moderate or medium amount	Significant amount	Large/excessive amount
0	0.5	1.5	3.5-4.0	4.0 and higher	8.0

According to research on the correlation between ketosis and weight loss, the ideal spot for losing weight is between 1.5-3.0. These figures represent the presence of ketones in the blood in mmol/L. Between 15-622 mg/dL is the preferred or recommended range for weight loss. While ketosis is beneficial for weight loss, especially if this state is reached and maintained for a length of time, moving into a state of autophagy may require a longer period of time, with intermittent fasting included, in order to exhaust the glucose in the body.

Intermittent Fasting

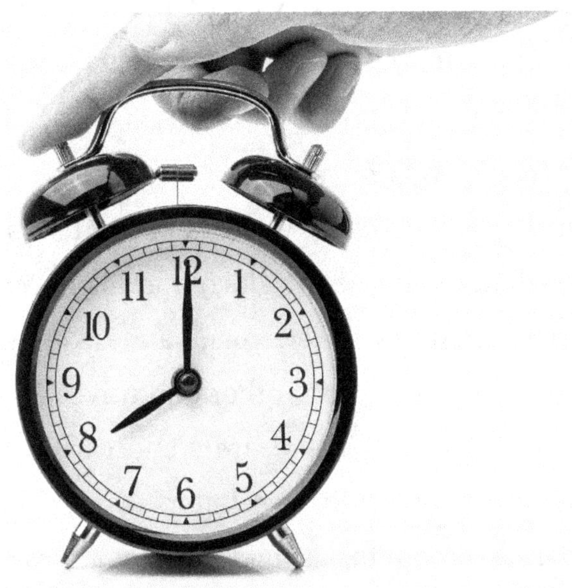

Intermittent fasting is becoming increasingly more common as studies show a lot of benefits from short-term fasts in between cycles of regular eating. When most people consider fasting, long-term avoidance of food and water for long periods of time, even days, may come to mind. While long-term fasting, for 24 hours or more, can be very beneficial, it is not recommended for everyone and should be a goal worked towards on a gradual, careful basis by trying shorter periods of time. While intermittent fasting denotes smaller periods of time, there are variations in the number of hours allocated between fasting, and feasting. For example, in a typical day, we may eat from

7:00 am, starting with breakfast, followed by lunch, a snack and dinner around 6 or 7 pm, our window would effectively be 12 hours, from 7 to 7, otherwise known as 12:12. The 12:12 refers to a 12-hour window to eat and the remaining 12 hours is fasting, for a total of one day, or 24 hours.

The Basics of Fasting

During a fast, drinking water is permitted, as well as any liquid that will not increase the glucose levels in your body. Acceptable options include water, tea, and coffee (with no sugar, sweeteners, milk or other additives), and sparkling or carbonated water. There are some carbonated beverages that have low or no-carb sweeteners, which may be included in moderate amounts, as they will not have an impact on the fasting process. Bone broth is sometimes consumed during a fast, though the opinions vary on whether this is recommended. Some experts will advise against it, as bone broth contains minerals and ingredients that essentially "break" a fast, though others recommend it as a way to continually get nutrients while enjoying all the benefits of a fast. The variance in opinion hinges on whether adding the broth is significant enough to impede the progress of fasting, or if it may enhance its potential.

For the purposes of autophagy, consuming anything, including water during a fast, can slow down the progression towards the production of autophagosomes, even if slightly. For this reason, it's often suggested to minimize water and liquids, or simply "dry" fast, which refers to avoiding all foods and drinks. Why do small or moderate amounts of liquids slow down the onset of autophagy? This is because our bodies will use anything that becomes available to use for repairing and building new cells and tissues, including the properties of water. While this is a small amount, and will not stop autophagy from occurring, especially during longer fasting periods, avoidance of all liquids is an option to clear the path towards achieving autophagy much sooner.

Different Types of Fasting

Each plan for intermittent fasting is divided into "windows" to identify when eating is permitted or when it is abstained from. A "fasting" window indicates fasting is in progress, and no food or drink is consumed. There are some exceptions that may be considered, which will be covered in this section, following the fasting methods. During the eating of feeding "window," food and drink are permitted as per your own way of eating, whether there are no changes made at all, or a new diet is started, such as ketogenic or low-calorie plan. If you decide to make significant changes to your diet, in conjunction with intermittent fasting, it's best to begin one plan first to get accustomed to it, before adding more changes. For example, begin eating low carb foods and reducing the overall carbohydrates and sugar in our diet, prior to adding periods of fasting. Alternatively, you can begin adjusting your schedule to intermittent fasting windows, gradually increasing the fasting window until you find a plan that works best, followed by changing your diet within each eating window.

The most advantageous aspect of intermittent fasting, which focus on when to eat, rather than what to eat, is the way it can be individualized to fit within your schedule for work, eating and rest. Although intermittent fasting does not specify which types of foods or diet to eat, adapting to and maintaining a low carb diet with wholesome foods is strongly recommended for best results. Combining the ketogenic diet with intermittent fasting, for example, while not a requirement, is often done to maximize the results of both ways of eating. This plan may also bring about autophagy more quickly than intermittent fasting without low carb eating, as glucose is already significantly reduced during eating hours. The following types of intermittent fasting plans are recommended in the following order:

12:12 Fasting Method: For Beginners

This is the easiest intermittent fasting plan, to begin with, as it will "train" or adapt your body and mind to the idea of timing your meals and eating within a specified window of hours or timeframe. The 12:12 method is realistic for people with no prior experience, as it is compatible with most regular daily eating schedules and eating routines. Planning this starter-fast option is as easy as choosing when to begin and stop each fasting and eating window:

<u>12:12 Plan A:</u>

This fasting plan begins on a Sunday evening after 7 pm, with the fasting "window" or period during which there is no food or drink, and ending the following morning at 7 am, when breakfast is served.

Day of the week	Sunday	Monday	Tuesday	Wednesday	Thursday	Friday	Saturday
Feeding or eating window	7 am to 7 pm (dinner is between 6-7 pm)	7 am to 7 pm	7 am to 7 pm	7 am to 7 pm	7 am to 7 pm	7 am to 7 pm	7 am to 7 pm
Fasting window	7 pm to 7 am the next morni	7 pm to 7 am the next mor	7 pm to 7 am the next mor	7 pm to 7 am the next morning	7 pm to 7 am the next morn	7 pm to 7 am the next mor	7 pm to 7 am the next mor

	ng	ning	ning		ing	ning	ning

This plan provides a generous window of eating between the daytime hours of 7 am to 7 pm, allowing more than enough time to enjoy breakfast, lunch, and dinner with periods of drinking and/or snacks in between. When fasting begins after 7 pm, no eating will occur until breakfast the following day, which begins at 7 am or later. The fasting hours or "window" can include sleeping, and usually does, as it makes the plan easier to follow and most people would not eat during the night. Another option for this plan, depending on your individual schedule, may look like plan B:

<u>12:12 Plan B:</u>

Day of the week	Sunday	Monday	Tuesday	Wednesday	Thursday	Friday	Saturday
Feeding or eating window	5am to 5pm (dinner is between 4-5 pm or skipped	5am to 5pm	5am to 5pm	5am to 5pm	5am to 5pm	5am to 5pm	5am to 5pm

	altoget her)						
Fastin g windo w	5pm to 5am the next morni ng	5pm to 5am the next mor ning	5pm to 5am the next mor ning	5pm to 5am the next morni ng	5pm to 5am the next morn ing	5pm to 5am the next mor ning	5pm to 5am the next mor ning

The second plan, which includes a fasting window of 5pm to 5am, is best suited to someone with an early start, providing a better opportunity to fit more meals earlier into the day while starting the fast at 5pm. This shift in hours, compared to the 7 to 7 plans in plan A, is a good fit for a meal plan that includes a large breakfast and lunch, with the option for a snack, and either no dinner or a light meal just prior to 5pm. The third option (below) is a good option for beginning the eating window later in the day if it is preferred to skip or delay breakfast for a brunch or early lunch.

12:12 Plan C:

Day of the week	Sunda y	Mon day	Tues day	Wedne sday	Thur sday	Frida y	Satur day
Feedi	12 pm	12	12	12 pm	12	12	12

ng or eating window	to 12am (breakfast is either skipped or shifted later or as an early lunch)	pm to 12am	pm to 12am	to 12am	pm to 12am	pm to 12am	pm to 12am
Fasting window	12am to 12 pm the following day	12am to 12 pm the following day	12am to 12 pm the following day	12am to 12 pm the following day	12am to 12 pm the following day	12am to 12 pm the following day	12am to 12 pm the following day

The later fasting window beginning at 12 pm until 12am provides later options for meals and works well for people who do not wish to include breakfast in their daily plan, and instead, shift their lunch and dinner meals later, leaving an option for a later snack before 12am. This plan also works well for people who work and/or go to bed late.

The 12:12 intermittent fasting plan will not get you into ketosis, nor will it accomplish a state of autophagy, unless food during the eating window is severely restricted, which is not recommended until you are ready for a longer fast, which will bring about both ketosis and autophagy. The benefits of this method lie in the following principles, which are established during the beginning of this plan for further success:

- Establishing a routine. If you haven't planned your meals before, intermittent fasting will give you definite time limits, so that you learn to work within these windows and budget your meals accordingly. While there is flexibility within each eating window, your meals are restricted within these hours.

- Individualizing your plan. If you have a busy schedule, planning your eating and fasting windows should be done with careful consideration of when you normally eat and/or when you desire to take your meals. Your schedule doesn't need to be etched in stone or planned for months in advance; you can shift your eating and fasting hours on a weekly or bi-weekly basis if it suits your schedule for work and other priorities.

- There are no dietary restrictions during intermittent

fasting unless you choose to implement them, or otherwise already restrict certain foods, calories or carbs in your diet. The focus is on when to eat and expanding the fasting window will automatically keep your caloric intake and total carbs lower during the fasting hours.

Once you have adapted to a 12:12 diet, the next step is to expand the fasting window and reducing the time frame for meals. The 16:8 is recommended for this option.

16:8 Intermittent Fasting Plan

The 16:8 method refers to an intermittent fasting schedule of 16 hours fasting and 8 hours of eating. While sixteen hours may seem like a long period of time, it is a good start for beginners, or the next step after adjusting to a 12:12 fasting plan. The 16:8 plan allows for a 16-hour fasting window, followed by an 8-hour eating window. Eating within 8 hours may seem like a far cry from 12 hours, though with a few minor adjustments, it is easy to adjust to within one or two weeks. Adjusting your meals from a 12-hour window to an 8-hour window can be as simple as shifting the same meals closer together or reducing the size and/or amount of meals. For example, if you skip a meal to fit your eating plan into a smaller time frame, add an extra light snack or simply reduce one or more of the meals, so they can be enjoyed closer together.

What does a 16:8 intermittent fasting plan look like? It can vary considerably, depending on your schedule. Like the 12:12 plan, you can begin early in the day, or later, to reflect when you wish to begin the eating window.

<u>16:8 Plan A:</u>

This fasting plan begins on a Sunday evening after 3 pm, with the fasting "window" or time period during which there is no food or drink, and ending the following morning at 7 am, when breakfast is served.

Day of the week	Sunday	Monday	Tuesday	Wednesday	Thursday	Friday	Saturday
Feeding or eating window	7 am to 3 pm (skip dinner or have a light snack)	7 am to 3 pm	7 am to 3 pm	7 am to 3 pm	7 am to 3 pm	7 am to 3 pm	7 am to 3 pm
Fasting window	3 pm to 7 am the next morni	3 pm to 7 am the next mor	3 pm to 7 am the next mor	3 pm to 7 am the next morning	3 pm to 7 am the next morn	3 pm to 7 am the next mor	3 pm to 7 am the next mor

	ng	ning	ning		ing	ning	ning

This fasting plan can work with three traditional meals: breakfast between 7-8 am, lunch at 11:30-12:30 and a light dinner or snack between 2-3 pm. Dinner can be omitted in place of a snack, or skipped altogether, if lunch is shifted to a later time, and a snack added between breakfast and lunch (mid-morning). If you tend to eat lighter meals, the 16:8 plan allows for as many as possible within the 8-hour eating window, as no food is taken during the fast.

<u>16:8 Plan B:</u>

This schedule is a variation on the 16:8 plan, which allows for a more substantial lunch and dinner, with a skipped breakfast for meal replacement in the late morning. Beginning the fasting window later in the date is an appropriate option for people who tend to skip breakfast as a habit, or prefer it later, mid-morning or skip directly to lunch for the first meal. If you have a large dinner the evening before, this can provide more sustenance until the next late morning or lunch hour.

Day of the week	Sunday	Monday	Tuesday	Wednesday	Thursday	Friday	Saturday
Feeding or eating	11 am to 7 pm	11 am to 7	11 am to 7	11 am to 7 pm	11 am to 7 pm	11 am to 7	11 am to 7

window	(skip breakfast or have late morning)	pm	pm			pm	pm
Fasting window	7 pm to 11 am the next morning	7 pm to 11 am the next morning	7 pm to 11 am the next morning	7 pm to 11 am the next morning	7 pm to 11 am the next morning	7 pm to 11 am the next morning	7 pm to 11 am the next morning

The 8-hour eating window resembles a standard working day or shift, which is usually between 7.5 to 8 hours each day. If you plan your eating hours just before and after work, and one or two opportunities in between, it leaves the remainder of the 24 hours as a fasting period. If you work, attend a school or other activities for an 8-hour period, the measuring process is easy and can be matched to either coincide with or overlap your eating window. If you have the type of employment that doesn't provide a lot of time to take breaks or eat, you may want to shift the hours earlier or later to accommodate.

<u>16:8 Plan C:</u>

In keeping with the 8-hour fasting window, the hours can be easily moved to start later, skipping breakfast with the option of moving lunch later as well, and focusing on eating later in the day, which results in breaking the fast later the following morning. This plan is ideal for people who generally start later in the day or wish to begin their eating window later. It allows for a late lunch and dinner, with a snack option in between:

Day of the week	Sunday	Monday	Tuesday	Wednesday	Thursday	Friday	Saturday
Feeding or eating window	1 pm to 9 pm (skip breakfast and shift lunch and dinner later)	1 pm to 9 pm	1 pm to 9 pm	1 pm to 9 pm	1 pm to 9 pm	1 pm to 9 pm	1 pm to 9 pm
Fasting	9 pm to 1	9 pm to 1	9 pm to 1	9 pm to 1	9 pm to 1	9 pm to 1	9 pm to 1

windo w	pm the next day	pm the next day	pm the next day	pm the next day	pm the next day	pm the next day	pm the next day

Aside from the suggested windows for eating and fasting for both the 12:12 and 16:8 plans, further adjustments can be made, provided that the consistency in adhering to the fasting window remains. For example, eating from 3 pm to 11 pm is acceptable and recommended if you work late hours, though it is important to stick with the fasting period of 11 pm to 3 pm the following day.

18:6 Intermittent Fasting Plan

The 18:6 plan is a minor shift from the 16:8 plan, and an easy one to switch to, once you've become comfortable with 16-hour fasts. It requires an additional 2 hours of fasting, which can simply be added to the end or beginning of your current schedule, or with one hour added onto each end of the window. This plan reduces the eating window to six hours, which essentially eliminates one of the three traditional meals. In order to adjust to this shorter time frame for meals, it may be beneficial to have three light meals within the six hours than two larger ones. This will provide more coverage during this window.

The 18-hour fast brings your body closer to reaching a state of ketosis, especially if your meals during the six hours are low carb and low glucose. During a fast, you will naturally become depleted in carbohydrates, which also moves you towards autophagy. While there is a variance in how and when autophagy is reached, as it varies depending on each individual, it can begin around 18 hours for some people and require a longer period of fasting for others. For this reason, this plan can be yet another stepping-stone towards a longer fast in the future.

18:6 Plan A:

This fasting plan begins on a Sunday evening after 1 pm, with the fasting "window" or time period during which there is no food or drink, and ending the following morning at 7 am, when breakfast is served.

Day of the week	Sunday	Monday	Tuesday	Wednesday	Thursday	Friday	Saturday
Feeding or eating window	7 am to 1 pm (includes breakfast with	7 am to 1 pm	7 am to 1 pm	7 am to 1 pm	7 am to 1 pm	7 am to 1 pm	7 am to 1 pm

	option s mid-morni ng snack and lunch)						
Fastin g windo w	1 pm to 7 am the next morni ng	1 pm to 7 am the next mor ning	1 pm to 7 am the next mor ning	1 pm to 7 am the next morni ng	1 pm to 7 am the next morn ing	1 pm to 7 am the next mor ning	1 pm to 7 am the next mor ning

An early start is a good option for this plan, concentrating the meals within the first six hours of the day. If you begin your working day later, eating highly nutritious meals within this time frame will provide a good source of fuel, allowing the body to seek sources of stored fats and other options once the energy is used from the previous meals.

In general, it is best to increase the nutrient density of your foods as your eating window shrinks, as there is a longer time period between meals once the fasting begins. While there are no specific meal plans for standard intermittent fasting, keeping the carbs and sugars low, while the protein, healthy fats and nutrients are high, will give your body and cells all that is needed to function well during a fasting window.

<u>18:6 Plan B:</u>

This fasting plan begins on a Sunday evening after 4 pm, allowing for a later start time the following morning at 10 am. A mid-morning beginning provides for a late breakfast or mid-morning snack to break the fast, followed by a standard lunch between 12-1 pm and a light dinner or healthy snack between 3-4 pm.

Day of the week	Sunday	Monday	Tuesday	Wednesday	Thursday	Friday	Saturday
Feeding or eating window	10 am to 4 pm (mid-morning snack, lunch and early dinner 3-4	10 am to 4 pm	10 am to 4 pm	10 am to 4 pm	10 am to 4 pm	10 am to 4 pm	10 am to 4 pm

	pm)						
Fastin g windo w	4 pm to 10 am the next morni ng	4 pm to 10 am the next mor ning	4 pm to 10 am the next mor ning	4 pm to 10 am the next morni ng	4 pm to 10 am the next morn ing	4 pm to 10 am the next mor ning	4 pm to 10 am the next mor ning

Once you adapt to shorter eating windows, the rules of breakfast, lunch, and dinner can be eliminated. For the purpose of following an easy plan, mid-morning, mid-afternoon and/or snack options are referenced in plans with shorter windows for eating. These can be considered by their traditional meal names, especially if they are taken around these times, though with intermittent fasting eating windows of 6 hours or less, usually one meal is skipped altogether in order to "fit" within the time frame.

<u>18:6 Plan C:</u>

This fasting plan begins on a Sunday evening after 7 pm, following a hearty dinner, with a breaking of the fast the following afternoon at or shortly after 1 pm. This is the perfect plan for skipping breakfast within the 6-hour window while maintaining two traditional meals (lunch and dinner). A mid-afternoon snack between 3-4 pm, followed by dinner between

6-7 pm works well within this plan. Lunch can be taken anytime after 1 pm.

Day of the week	Sunday	Monday	Tuesday	Wednesday	Thursday	Friday	Saturday
Feeding or eating window	1 pm to 7 pm (lunch, mid-afternoon snack, late dinner)	1 pm to 7 pm	1 pm to 7 pm	1 pm to 7 pm	1 pm to 7 pm	1 pm to 7 pm	1 pm to 7 pm
Fasting window	7 pm to 1 pm the next morning	7 pm to 1 pm the next morning	7 pm to 1 pm the next morning	7 pm to 1 pm the next morning	7 pm to 1 pm the next morning	7 pm to 1 pm the next morning	7 pm to 1 pm the next morning

Many people prefer to stay with the 18:6 plan, as it provides a beneficial weight-loss plan. It may or may not provide a path to autophagy or ketosis, depending on the types of foods consumed during the eating window. To reach autophagy, the best option is to expand the fasting window, when it is comfortable to so. This can be a gradual shift from six to five hours a day, for a 19:5 plan, then moving to 20:4, which is the next milestone.

20:4 Intermittent Fasting Plan

The 20:4 fasting plan is often the option many people choose before "jumping" into a full 24-hour fast. As with all fasting methods, take it gradually until you reach this stage, as a 20-hour fast can be a significant change for many. This plan essentially reduces the eating window to four hours, which provides a few options: focus on one meal and supplement with a smaller, lighter meal, or enjoy two full meals at the very beginning of the eating window, and another towards the last half hour. Regardless of how this plan is approached, it greatly reduces meal options, which makes planning a major factor in success.

On a positive note, a 20-hour fast can bring the onset of autophagy for some people. The two-hour increase from an 18-hour fast to 20 hours can be significant in this stage, as autophagy usually begins anywhere between 18-24 hours, which is also a variable and highly contingent on each individual eating plan. Within this range of time, there is a "peak" period where ketosis and autophagy are at their most effective state.

Another advantage of the four-hour plan is the versatility in when to begin and end the eating window. This plan can be switched weekly or every 2-3 weeks to adjust according to preference and schedule. If you have a special occasion or other event planned, including a vacation, shifting the 4-hour window to a later time frame to capture a special meal is available. For the first sample plan below, the four hours begin early in the day, to focus on getting the most out of nutrients and food early for the remainder of the day, and throughout the fasting window:

<u>20:4 Plan A:</u>

This fasting plan begins late Sunday morning and lasts until the following morning at 7 am. The focus on this plan is on a nutrient-rich, high energy meal and supplement within the morning hours, so that there is a good amount of sustenance for the remainder of the day, during the fasting window. The focus for this plan on breakfast, with a mid-morning option for a supplement or snack. To avoid hunger pangs early into the fasting window, breakfast can be taken later, between 10-11 am, and a light snack between 7-7:30am.

Day of the week	Sunday	Monday	Tuesday	Wednesday	Thursday	Friday	Saturday
Feeding or	7 am to 11	7 am to 11	7 am to 11	7 am to 11	7 am to 11	7 am to 11	7 am to 11

eating window	am (includes breakfast with options mid-morning snack)	am	am	am	am	am	am
Fasting window	1 pm to 7 am the next morning	1 pm to 7 am the next morning	1 pm to 7 am the next morning	1 pm to 7 am the next morning	1 pm to 7 am the next morning	1 pm to 7 am the next morning	1 pm to 7 am the next morning

This plan can be slightly adjusted to begin earlier, at 5 or 6 am, and ending four hours later, at 9 or 10 am.

<u>20:4 Plan B:</u>

This fasting plan begins mid-afternoon on Sunday, ending the following day in the late morning. An early 4-hour window, as illustrated in 20:4 plan A may be too restrictive for many people, who wish to include a later meal before starting the fast.

Day of the week	Sunday	Monday	Tuesday	Wednesday	Thursday	Friday	Saturday
Feeding or eating window	10 am to 2 pm (includes breakfast or mid-morning snack with lunch)	10 am to 2 pm	10 am to 2 pm	10 am to 2 pm	10 am to 2 pm	10 am to 2 pm	10 am to 2 pm
Fasting window	2 pm to 10 am the next morning	2 pm to 10 am the next morning	2 pm to 10 am the next morning	2 pm to 10 am the next morning	2 pm to 10 am the next morning	2 pm to 10 am the next morning	2 pm to 10 am the next morning

The most beneficial aspect of this plan is the inclusion of both breakfast and lunch if desired. This schedule is also an option to one full meal, plus a lighter meal with an additional supplement. During this shorter eating window, it's strongly recommended to eat protein and fat-rich foods that can provide fuel over the next day. Breaking a fast after a window is completed may tempt some people to overeat. This can be avoided by planning and preparing a meal that will digest slowly, such as lean meats, tofu or tempeh and dark green vegetables high in iron and protein (all of which contain fiber). Unless your diet consists of low carb foods only, there is the option of including whole fruits and/or vegetables high in carbs, but also high in potassium and fiber, which offset the effects that carbohydrates have on the body. This fuel will be used up quickly during the fasting window. Examples of healthy foods that contain moderately high carbohydrates include sweet potatoes, bananas, and cherries.

<u>20:4 Plan C:</u>

The third sample option for fasting four hours each day begins at lunch until close to dinner. There is an option of including lunch and skipping dinner for a mid-afternoon snack or splitting two smaller, equal-sized meals within the eating window.

Day	Sund	Mond	Tues	Wedne	Thurs	Frida	Satur
of	ay	ay	day	sday	day	y	day

the week							
Feeding or eating window	12 pm to 4 pm (includes lunch or early afternoon snack with dinner)	12 pm to 4 pm	12 pm to 4 pm	12 pm to 4 pm	12 pm to 4 pm	12 pm to 4 pm	12 pm to 4 pm
Fasting window	4 pm to 12 pm the next afternoon	4 pm to 12 pm the next afternoon	4 pm to 12 pm the next afternoon	4 pm to 12 pm the next afternoon	4 pm to 12 pm the next afternoon	4 pm to 12 pm the next afternoon	4 pm to 12 pm the next afternoon

The focus of this window, from 12-4 pm, can be placed on lunch as the main meal, with a supplement or light early dinner meal between 3-4 pm. Once the fasting window begins at 4 pm, eating a good amount of healthy, whole foods within the four hours will give you enough to sustain your body with nutrients until the following day at noon. Even where your body becomes low on fuel, which will occur during ketosis, and during autophagy, including all the daily nutrient requirements within the four hours is essential to providing your body with a healthy start before fasting begins.

20:4 Plan D:

The final sample option for fasting four hours each day begins after lunch and focuses on the traditional dinner time for the main meal of the day. This plan can implement a hearty meal between 4-6, followed by a lighter, healthy snack between 7-8 pm. Since this eating window starts very late into the day, it's a recommended plan for people who sleep late and begin their day either later in the morning or towards the afternoon. One example of people who will benefit are shift workers or those who generally work evenings or later hours.

Day of the week	Sunday	Monday	Tuesday	Wednesday	Thursday	Friday	Saturday
Feeding or eating	4 pm to 8 pm	4 pm to 8 pm	4 pm to 8 pm	4 pm to 8 pm	4 pm to 8 pm	4 pm to 8 pm	4 pm to 8 pm

window	(includes lunch or early afternoon snack with dinner)						
Fasting window	8 pm to 4 pm the next day	8 pm to 4 pm the next day	8 pm to 4 pm the next day	8 pm to 4 pm the next day	8 pm to 4 pm the next day	8 pm to 4 pm the next day	8 pm to 4 pm the next day

Considering all four of the sample plans, and any number of variations in between, changes can be easily shifted to adjust from one plan to another where it is most suitable. A rotating schedule of different plans may also work for some people, such as 4-8 pm for week one, followed by 12-4 pm for week two, and so on. Most people will adjust to the four-hour fast within a week, though working towards a 6-hour or 8-hour eating window is the best strategy before starting a four-hour window, and especially before diving into a full day or 24-hour fast.

24-Hour Fasting Plan

The full-day fast is an ideal way to reach your autophagy goal, and it is a powerful way to lose weight and maintain consistent weight management on an ongoing basis. While it may seem like an extreme fasting method, it is not recommended for everyone; consulting a doctor or medical professional should be done before starting this method. To plan for the 24-hour fasting window, take into consideration the following:

- Fasting for a full 24 hours should be done only twice or three times weekly at the most. During regular meal planning in between full-day fasts, make sure you include as many whole, healthy foods as possible.

- If you feel faint or weak at any point during a fast, whether it is a duration of 24 hours or less, make sure to have some water and contact a health professional if you have a medical condition that may be impacted by fasting. If needed, break the fast with a light snack and drink some water.

- Drink plenty of water to ensure you have enough hydration during the fast. There is another method of fasting called "dry" fasting, which is more restrictive and does not include any liquid, including water. While dry fasting can be particularly effective in beginning autophagy, it is best to practice in shorter time frames before extending to one full day, so that your body becomes accustomed to the effects of abstaining from food and water.

- Get plenty of rest. This applies to all forms of fasting. A good night's sleep is essential in using your body's nutrient stores for important building and repairs to your brain, cells, and tissues.

<u>24-Hour Fasting (Two days a week): Plan A</u>

To begin your first 24-hour fasting plan, try just two days each week. This may seem like a different path from the 18:6, 20:4 daily intermittent fasting plans that precede this one, though taking a full day off from food consumption should not be taken lightly. The first sample option, below, designates two days for a full 24-hour fast: day 1 as Sunday and day 2 as Wednesday. The positioning of these days allows for equal distribution between both fasting days, allowing for 2-3 days of regular eating in between.

Day of the week	Sunday	Monday	Tuesday	Wednesday	Thursday	Friday	Saturday
Fasting	Fasting from	Break fast	Regular	Fasting from	Break fast	Regular	Regular

and/or eating window (24 hours)	9 am until the next day (Day 1 of fasting)	at 9am for breakfast	eating	9 am until the next day (Day 2 of fasting)	at 9am for breakfast	eating	eating

Options for this plan include shifting the hours to different start and end times. Plan A allows for breakfast prior to 9am before beginning the fast, with a breaking of the fast the following day after 9am. If you begin work earlier than 9am during the week, the start and end time for the fasting window can be moved earlier to 7 or 8am. The same can be done for a later start time, as illustrated in the second sample, plan B.

<u>24-Hour Fasting (Two days a week): Plan B</u>

In the second sample, the two fasting days are altered to begin at lunch, allowing for more time in the morning for a full breakfast, with the option of a light mid-morning snack before beginning a fast at 12 noon. On the following day, the fast is broken at the same time for lunch. This works well with more schedules, as lunch doesn't fluctuate as much as breakfast, which can be anywhere from 5am to 9am for many people, while lunch tends to center around noon.

Day of the week	Sunday	Monday	Tuesday	Wednesday	Thursday	Friday	Saturday
Fasting and/or eating window (24 hours)	Fasting from 12 pm until the next day (Day 1 of fasting)	Breakfast at 12 pm for lunch	Regular eating	Fasting from 12 pm, following breakfast until the next day (Day 2 of fasting)	Breakfast at 12 pm for lunch	Regular eating	Regular eating

A 24-hour, twice-weekly fasting schedule can be increased to three days a week, as long as a full day of regular eating is scheduled in between each fasting day: for each 24-hour fasting period, there should be a minimum of 24 hours of regular eating following the full day fast.

<u>24-Hour Fasting (Three days a week): Plan C</u>

Three 24-hour days of fasting will give you more opportunities to benefit from autophagy on a more regular basis while getting the most out of ketosis during the fasting days.

Day of the week	Sunday	Monday	Tuesday	Wednesday	Thursday	Friday	Saturday
Fasting and/or eating window (24 hours)	Fasting from 12 pm until the next day (Day 1 of fasting)	Breakfast at 12 pm for lunch (regular eating resumes for 24 hours until the	Fasting from 12 pm, following breakfast until the next day (Day 2 of fasting)	Breakfast at 12 pm for lunch	Regular eating	Fasting from 12 pm, following breakfast until the next day (Day 3 of fasting)	Breakfast at 12 pm for lunch (regular eating resumes for 24 hours until the next day)

		next day)					

This sample plan starts at 12 pm, three times a week. Due to the seven days each week, there may be an extra day in between two of the fasting days, with exactly 24 hours of regular eating in between the others. The first day of fasting, day 1, begins after 12 pm on Sunday, with a break the following day, Monday, after 12. A period of 24 hours begins from 12 pm on Monday until the following day at 12 pm, when the second day of fasting begins and ends on Wednesday at 12 pm. Thursday remains a regular eating day with no fasting. Friday begins the third day or 24 hours of fasting at 12 pm, which breaks the following day at 12 pm, leaving another 24 hours of regular eating until the next fasting period, which begins on the following Sunday at 12 pm.

The two-day or three-day 24-hour fasts can be adjusted to accommodate any schedule, provided a minimum 24 hours of regular eating is scheduled in between each fasting day. While this plan is an excellent way to reach the goal of autophagy, there are two more options that may be considered for either autophagy and/or dietary reasons: alternative day fasting and the 5:2 method.

Alternate Day Fasting

This intermittent fasting method takes the two or three days per week approach and increases the frequency of fasting to every other day, alternating one day of regular eating with one day of fasting, 24 hours for each period. This pattern can be done on a short-term or longer-term basis, provided you have enough nutrients and eat healthy, whole foods with little or no processing or artificial additives. The necessity of implementing healthier, more sustainable foods becomes increasingly more important as fasting windows and frequency expands.

The schedule below provides a guide on how alternate day fasting looks like and how it can be implemented into your regular schedule. The first plan works with the 12 pm to 12 pm option, as offered in the weekly 24-hour fasting samples, and is a good time frame to begin with, as it ensures that you will have at least one meal each day, either before or after 12 pm, depending on which day(s) you start and end each fasting window. Due to the nature of alternate fasting, where every other day of the week will vary from the first to the second week, this plan is shown in a span of two weeks:

Alternate Day Fasting: Plan A

Day of the week (Week 1)	Sunday	Monday	Tuesday	Wednesday	Thursday	Friday	Saturday
Fasti	Fasti	Brea	Fasti	Breakf	Fasti	Breakf	Fasti

ng and/ or eatin g wind ow (24 hour s)	ng from 12 pm until the next day (Day 1 of fastin g)	kfast at 12 pm for lunch (regu lar eatin g resu mes for 24 hours until the next day)	ng from 12 pm, follo wing brea kfast until the next day (Day 2 of fastin g)	ast at 12 pm for lunch (regul ar eating resum es for 24 hours until the next day)	ng from 12 pm, follo wing break fast until the next day (Day 3 of fastin g)	ast at 12 pm for lunch (regul ar eating resum es for 24 hours until the next day)	ng from 12 pm, follo wing break fast until the next day (Day 4 of fastin g)
Day of the week (Wee k 2)	Sund ay	Mon day	Tues day	Wedne sday	Thur sday	Friday	Satur day
Fasti	Brea	Fasti	Brea	Fastin	Brea	Fastin	Break

ng and/ or eatin g wind ow (24 hour s)	kfast at 12 pm for lunch (regu lar eatin g resu mes for 24 hour s until the next day)	ng from 12 pm, follo wing break fast until the next day (Day 5 of fastin g)	kfast at 12 pm for lunch (regu lar eatin g resu mes for 24 hour s until the next day)	g from 12 pm, followi ng breakf ast until the next day (Day 6 of fasting)	kfast at 12 pm for lunch (regu lar eatin g resu mes for 24 hour s until the next day)	g from 12 pm, follow ing breakf ast until the next day (Day 7 of fastin g) (Day 3 of fastin g)	fast at 12 pm for lunch (regul ar eatin g resu mes for 24 hours until the next day)

The fasting days over a 14-day or two-week period are scheduled as follows:

- Sunday (day 1, week 1)
- Tuesday (day 3, week 1)
- Thursday (day 5, week 1)

- Saturday (day 7, week 1)
- Monday (day 9, week 2)
- Wednesday (day 11, week 2)
- Friday (day 13, week 2)

On day 14th, or Saturday, the final day of the two weeks, regular eating is resumed at 12 pm, with fasting beginning on the following day at 12 pm as per the first week's schedule. Rotating the two weeks to accommodate alternate days of fasting with eating can be adjusted to begin on either the first or second day of week one and follow accordingly. The next plan provides an earlier start time to allow for an earlier breakfast.

<u>Alternate Day Fasting: Plan B</u>

Day of the week (Week 1)	Sunday	Monday	Tuesday	Wednesday	Thursday	Friday	Saturday
Fasting and/or eating wind	Fasting from 8am until the next	Breakfast at 8am for breakfast	Fasting from 8am, following brea	Breakfast at 8am for breakfast (regul	Fasting from 8am, following wing break	Breakfast at 8am for breakfast (regul	Fasting from 8am, following wing break

ow (24 hours)	day (Day 1 of fasting)	(regular eating resumes for 24 hours until the next day)	kfast until the next day (Day 2 of fasting)	ar eating resumes for 24 hours until the next day)	fast until the next day (Day 3 of fasting)	ar eating resumes for 24 hours until the next day)	fast until the next day (Day 4 of fasting)
Day of the week (Week 2)	Sunday	Monday	Tuesday	Wednesday	Thursday	Friday	Saturday
Fasting and/or eating g	Breakfast at 8am for break	Fasting from 8am, following	Breakfast at 8am for brea	Fasting from 8am, following breakf	Breakfast at 8am for break	Fasting from 8am, following breakf	Breakfast at 8am for break

wind ow (24 hour s)	fast (regu lar eatin g resu mes for 24 hour s until the next day)	break fast until the next day (Day 5 of fastin g)	kfast (regu lar eatin g resu mes for 24 hour s until the next day)	ast until the next day (Day 6 of fasting)	fast (regu lar eatin g resu mes for 24 hour s until the next day)	ast until the next day (Day 7 of fastin g)	fast (regul ar eatin g resu mes for 24 hours until the next day)

The second sample plan follows the exact same idea as plan A, with a shift from 12 pm to 8am. This is an ideal method of fasting for schedules that require an earlier meal taken either before the fasting begins (before 8am) and once the window ends (just after 8am the following morning). The third and final option displays how a later start would look like over a two-week period, beginning at 4 pm.

<u>Alternate Day Fasting: Plan C</u>

Day of the week (Week 1)	Sunday	Monday	Tuesday	Wednesday	Thursday	Friday	Saturday
Fasting and/or eating window (24 hours)	Fasting from 4 pm until the next day (Day 1 of fasting)	Breakfast at 4 pm for dinner (regular eating resumes for 24 hours until the next	Fasting from 4 pm, following a late lunch or mid-afternoon snack until the next day (Day 2 of fastin	Breakfast at 4 pm for dinner (regular eating resumes for 24 hours until the next day)	Fasting from 4 pm, following a late lunch or mid-afternoon snack until the next day (Day 3 of fastin	Breakfast at 4 pm for dinner (regular eating resumes for 24 hours until the next day)	Fasting from 4 pm, following a late lunch or mid-afternoon snack until the next day (Day 4 of fastin

		day)	g)		g)		g)
Day of the week (Week 2)	Sunday	Monday	Tuesday	Wednesday	Thursday	Friday	Saturday
Fasting and/or eating window (24 hours)	Breakfast at 4 pm for dinner (regular eating resumes for 24 hours until the	Fasting from 4 pm, following a late lunch or mid-afternoon snack until the next day (Day 5 of	Breakfast at 4 pm for dinner (regular eating resumes for 24 hours until the	Fasting from 4 pm, following a late lunch or mid-afternoon snack until the next day (Day 6 of fasting	Breakfast at 4 pm for dinner (regular eating resumes for 24 hours until the	Fasting from 4 pm, following a late lunch or mid-afternoon snack until the next day (Day 7 of	Breakfast at 4 pm for dinner (regular eating resumes for 24 hours until the next

	next day)	fastin g)	next day)	)	next day)	fastin g)	day)

All alternate day fasting samples are beneficial in the same way, with the only difference being preference and schedule. If alternating days becomes too much, changing back to twice a week for 24 hours or a 20:4 or 18:6 plan may be a better option. While intermittent fasting is beneficial for many people, it can present challenges for some and is not the best method for everyone.

Extended Fasting for Periods of Over 24 Hours

Once you have mastered 24-hour fasting and wish to extend your level of fast to yet another milestone, there are extended options of over 24 hours. Typically, this is done less frequently, to allow your body to recover from abstaining from food for over one day, or up to 3 days in total. Extended periods of fasting, if followed correctly, will provide the benefits of autophagy and ketosis within the first 24 hours. Any extension of the fasting period will continue the benefits of both, though the peak or desired point of maximum effectiveness for both ketosis and autophagy will decline after 24 hours. For this reason, fasting longer than 24 hours is not necessarily required, though it can provide additional health benefits, such as detoxification and significant weight loss within a short period of time. Once you are prepared to embark on a long fast of 30,

48 or 60 hours or more, plan to ensure you have a stress-free environment and support available before you begin:

- Speak to your family, friends, doctor, and/or anyone else who will be directly affected by your extended fast and may be able to provide support, encouragement, and/or advice.
- Rule out any medical conditions that may worsen or negatively impact your health during a long-term fast.
- Avoid beginning a fast during a stressful time or when there is a special occasion. It is during exceptional circumstances and event that we may want to break the fast and/or enjoy a meal that will occur during the fasting window.
- If you work a standard five days each week, Monday through Friday, plan an extended fast over a weekend to minimize temptation at work to eat
- Spend as much time as possible in a calming, natural environment to get the most out of the experience. Fasting shouldn't be considered a chore or unpleasant, but rather, a rest from eating and other activities that increase stress. If there is the option of spending a weekend away in the countryside or somewhere else natural and relaxing, this will greatly improve your chances of success.

- Keep a diary of your experience and take note of any sensations, side effects, or experiences of your fasting journey. This will help you to identify any concerns and/or challenges that can be addressed

- Exercise mindfully. High impact exercise is excellent for a regular dieting and short term fasting, though should be used with caution during extended periods of fasting. For this reason, begin slowly and gently, adding yoga, Pilates and/or other gently guided methods of stretching and moving that will keep your body fit while giving you more relaxation

- Get a massage. Every now and again, whether we have a health condition requiring massage therapy or not, it can be an excellent way to work through and minimize our body's stress, especially during periods of fasting.

How long should I fast? It depends on your goal. Athletes and people who tend to be very active will take a long fast, between 60-72 hours (up to three days) to maximize burning fat stores and losing weight fast, while continuing to exercise and build lean muscle mass. It is during this process where autophagy begins to break down old cellular matter, once all other sources of energy have been exhausted, in order to repair and rebuild in the body. This process makes our bodies more efficient, and just one reason why more athletes are implementing a fasting plan into their diet to gain the benefits of autophagy.

The chart below indicates how scheduling a 30-hour fast can take place over a period of two days, from Sunday at 12 pm until the following day, Monday, at 6pm. Since the 30-hour period is slightly longer than 24 hours, it may be possible to fast for this duration of time once per week, though once every 2-4 weeks is beneficial and allows for plenty of time to recover from the extended time frame.

<u>30-Hour Fasting Plan</u>

Day of the week	Sunday	Monday	Tuesday	Wednesday	Thursday	Friday	Saturday
Fasting period (over one day) and regular eatin	Fasting begins at 12 pm	Fasting until 6pm (completing a 30 hour fast)	Regular eating	Regular eating	Regular eating	Regular eating	Regular eating

g							

The next sample plan shows how a 48-hour or two full days of fasting may be scheduled during a regular week.

<u>48-Hour Fasting Plan</u>

Day of the week	Sunday	Monday	Tuesday	Wednesday	Thursday	Friday	Saturday
Fasting period (over one day) and regular eating	Fasting begins at 12 pm	Fasting continues	Fasting continues until 12 pm, completing a full 48 hours	Regular eating	Regular eating	Regular eating	Regular eating

The two-day fast begins similarly to the 30-hour fast, at noon or 12 pm on one day, continuing for the next day (Monday), then ending on Tuesday at 12 pm. A 48-hour fast should be done no more than once every two weeks, and preferably just once monthly. If you wish to benefit more often from fasting, it's best to implement smaller, more frequent intermittent fasting options before and after a long-term fast, allowing for one full day on either end (before and after) of the extended fast.

Increasing the fasting window longer, to 60 or 72 hours should not be done more than once a month. Extended fasting for any length of time after 24 hours should be done carefully to ensure that enough healthy foods are consumed just prior to and immediately following the fast. Breaking a fast, especially after a long-term session, should be done first with a light, easy to digest meal, to avoid any possible indigestion or other issues.

The following two plans, for 60 hours and 72 hours, indicate how these long-term fasts can be scheduled in a one-week time, though should only be done once every month or every two months:

<u>60-Hour Fasting Plan</u>

Day of the week	Sunday	Monday	Tuesday	Wednesday	Thursday	Friday	Saturday
Fasting period (over one	Fasting begins at 12 pm	Fasting continues	Fasting continues until 6pm,	Regular eating	Regular eating	Regular eating	Regular eating

day) and regular eating			completing a full 60 hours				

This 60-hour schedule provides a partial day of fasting beginning on Sunday, followed by a full day on Monday, with a break in fasting at dinner time on Tuesday. The fasting period is essentially two and a half days long.

72-Hour Fasting Plan

Day of the week	Sunday	Monday	Tuesday	Wednesday	Thursday	Friday	Saturday
Fasting period (over one day) and regular	Fasting begins at 12 pm	Fasting continues	Fasting continues	Fasting ends at lunch or 12 pm	Regular eating	Regular eating	Regular eating

eatin g							

The 72-hour fast, which is three full days, is the longest recommended fast. Any fasting for longer than three days can cause weakness and other symptoms, if not properly prepared for. While an extended fast can be rewarding, it also requires staying in tune with your body's needs and paying attention to any symptoms that may cause more harm than good. During your fast, take time for yourself to meditate, stretch, and rest in order to get the most out of this state. It's a time to reflect on your goals and reasons for fasting and taking comfort in the positive outcome.

Dry Fasting Versus Wet (or Regular) Fasting

During a fast, water and a limited amount of liquids that do not increase or affect your glucose levels, may be consumed as needed. The benefits of fasting will not be adversely affected by drinking water and other permissible liquids, and ketosis will be achieved in the exact same way with or without liquids. The reason for dry fasting is due to how much quickly cell regeneration can be achieved through autophagy, a state that is reached sooner when all foods and liquids are abstained from altogether. This form of fasting should be done with careful consideration to avoid dehydration. Dry fasting is practiced for religious and spiritual reasons, for short, intermittent periods or longer, expanded time frames. If you plan on dry fasting, any and all of the above intermittent fasting plans, including more extended periods apply. Start with a short time frame, and gradually increase over time, until you reach the desired plan to achieve your objective. Keep the following tips in mind when dry fasting:

- Avoid high impact exercise that will dehydrate the body quickly. While exercise of any kind is beneficial during a regular or "wet" fast, it should be limited if liquids are not consumed. Low impact movement, such as stretching and walking, are the best options during a dry fast

- Monitor how you feel, especially your energy levels. If you have the option of taking a day off work or minimizing your tasks for the day, it can provide a good opportunity to focus on the moment. At any time if you begin to feel weak or sick, sipping a bit of water may be an option to avoid getting ill. Usually, this is not an issue, and most people get through a dry fast with little to no problems. There will be some symptoms associated with feeling tired, hungry, and thirsty, though they are temporary and will come and go during the fasting window.

- Dry fasting is not for everyone. If you don't succeed the

first time, try again, or simply stick with other forms of fasting that allow for liquids and small periods of time.

5:2 Fasting Method

The 5:2 method is different than all other forms of fasting, in that it allows for some food consumption during the fasting window. This method consists of five days of regular eating and two days of fasting or consuming food and drink of up to 500 calories only. During the regular days, there are no carb or calorie restrictions, though eating low carb is an option. The two days of fasting are spread across the week, to ensure at least one full day of regular eating falls within both days.

The 5:2 fasting plan can vary from week to week, depending on personal preference and schedule. The advantage of this plan is the flexibility, and the allowance of some food and drink consumption during the fasting days. The following schedule is a sample of how this plan can be organized in a typical week:

5:2 Fasting Schedule: Plan A

Day of the week	Sun day	Monda y	Tues day	Wedn esday	Thur sday	Friday	Satur day
5:2 meth od (two	Reg ular eati ng	Fastin g (eating up to	Reg ular eati ng	Fastin g (eating up to	Regu lar eatin g	Regul ar eating	Regul ar eatin g

days fasting, 5 days regular eating)		500 calories for the day)		500 calories for the day)			

The above plan provides just one full day of regular eating in between the two fasting days of the week. The period in between these 500-calorie days can be expanded to two or three days, as shown in plan B and C:

<u>5:2 Fasting Schedule: Plan B</u>

Day of the week	Sunday	Monday	Tuesday	Wednesday	Thursday	Friday	Saturday
5:2 method (two days fasting, 5	Regular eating	Fasting (eating up to 500 calories for	Regular eating	Regular eating	Fasting (eating up to 500 calori	Regular eating	Regular eating

days regular eating)		the day)			es for the day)		

The second plan (above) allows for two days of regular eating in between fasting, while the third option provides three days in between during the week, with one fasting day on Sunday, and the other on a Thursday.

5:2 Fasting Schedule: Plan C

Day of the week	Sunday	Monday	Tuesday	Wednesday	Thursday	Friday	Saturday
5:2 method (two days fasting, 5 days regular	Fasting (eating up to 500 calories for the day)	Regular eating	Regular eating	Regular eating	Fasting (eating up to 500 calories for the day)	Regular eating	Regular eating

eatin g)						

Options for eating during the 500-calorie fasting days include simple foods that provide enough nutrients to supplement the carbs and fat stores your body already contains in order to use during the fasting window:

- One or two boiled eggs (for the duration of the day)
- Small or moderate green salad with a balsamic dressing. Cucumbers, shredded carrots, slivered almonds are among the options to include with spinach, arugula and/or lettuce.
- Bone broth and/or miso soup
- A small portion of fish (tuna or salmon) with salad
- Tea, coffee and lots of water
- Avoid all sugar and sweeteners as much as possible

While the 5:2 fasting method is very beneficial for weight loss and maintenance and reducing or preventing many health conditions and diseases, it's not the most effective method of achieving ketosis or autophagy. This is due to having no window where there is complete avoidance of all food, as in other intermittent or long-term fasting methods. While the body is consuming food, even in small amounts, reaching autophagy is not likely. The 5:2 fasting plan is a good option in between periods of intermittent fasting, where you decide to take a break from traditional fasting completely while keeping your food intake monitored for calories for weight maintenance.

Alternating Between Carb Cycling and Low Carb Eating

Bodybuilders and athletes may often choose to "carb-up" or increase the number of carbohydrates in their diet for certain periods of time, to prepare for marathons, races, and other very physically demanding activities. This may infrequently occur, only a few days or hours prior to such an event, or on an intermittent basis, to match a high impact exercise schedule on certain days, while reducing the carb intake for the remaining days to match lower impact exercise or rest periods. This type of carb "cycling" usually revolves around a ketogenic diet, with the low carb days strictly adhering to the 20 grams or below target, and the higher carb days are increasing to add more fuel for the activities. This type of diet is best suited for experienced athletes who are not looking to lose weight, but rather build muscle and maximize the amount of energy, whether it be carbs or fat, to use for that purpose.

Low to high carb cycling will not achieve autophagy, though once the carbs are fully depleted after a strenuous exercise event, moving into a mode of fasting instead of low carb eating can bring a period of ketosis and result in autophagy soon after. This is due to the body's need for materials to build more muscle and tissue. When food is restricted or abstained from for a period of 18 hours or more following a high carb day and depletion of those carbs as energy, autophagy can be easier to achieve at the 18-hour point. So, while this form of diet isn't the best way to reach autophagy, it can definitely lead to this if intermittent fasting is combined during the low carb part of the cycle.

Other Diets and Methods for Achieving Ketosis and Autophagy

Are there any specific diets and other ways of eating that achieve autophagy? While many paths lead to autophagy, there is no specific one-fits-all diet that will make it work for everyone in the same way. Like diets, not all methods of eating or meal plans work for the individual. For this reason, the ketogenic diet and low carb eating provide a method or way of eating, by reducing the number of carbohydrates, while increasing fats and protein, though without setting strict guidelines on the calories consumed or amount of foods. The ketogenic diet provides a head-start to intermittent fasting, which leads to autophagy, by reducing the carbohydrates in the body prior to fasting. This allows the body to use up its fat stores sooner during a fast and moving onto cell regeneration much sooner. A few points to keep in mind when planning for intermittent fasting that leads to autophagy:

- Become familiar with foods that are low in carbs and make them a regular part of your diet, even if you do not plan on committing to a ketogenic diet on a full-time basis; you can begin to restrict carbs on a gradual basis to prepare ahead.

- Drink water when you feel hungry. Most hunger pangs are symptoms of thirst, and drinking plenty of water will help reduce overeating as well as eating the wrong foods

- Stay active. Exercise and engage in regular movement to maintain and regulate your metabolism. It also keeps your body in an accelerated state of burning carbs, followed by fat stores, which is a quicker way to becoming fat-adapted, where your body switches into ketosis and burns fat as its main fuel. This is a good way to prepare for intermittent fasting and further towards autophagy.

Every person's body varies in response to intermittent fasting and the different types of diets that support ketosis and reducing carbs. Try different methods to determine which works best for your body and goals and avoid any methods that don't yield the results you want to achieve.

Chapter 5: The Horizon of Autophagy

Autophagy is a fascinating tool that we can switch on in our bodies to replenish and rejuvenate our cells, which are the basic building blocks of our body. Cells are continually dying and regenerating within our bodies, and as we age, the regeneration of cells slows down, where fewer cells are replacing the ones that die off. As a result, our body processes slow down as there are fewer cells to do the same work required to function. While increasing the number of cells is simply not possible or available, improving the quality of the fewer new cells that replace, the older ones, is paramount to maintaining excellent health and slowing down the aging process. Effectively, quality will take the place of quantity. With fewer cells, your body can continue to function exceptionally well, as long as only good quality cells and tissues develop on an ongoing basis.

At which point does autophagy occur? The first step is to determine at which point ketosis begins, which is the switch from burning carbs or glucose as fuel to stores of fat. When this occurs, your body is using up the fat as fuel because there are no carbs left to use. During this time, cellular repair and rebuilding are continually in process, and the body will find any sources possible to accomplish this goal. The chart below indicates the approximate decrease in plasma insulin in the body during various points of a fast, in increments of 6 hours, starting at twelve hours of fasting. According to the chart, insulin steadily decreases between 12 and 24 hours, from just above 60 to around 40 pmol/L of insulin. After 24 hours, the insulin levels begin to increase, in part due to the body's production of glucose. This occurs during ketosis when the body produces ketones in response to low glucose levels. From 24 hours to 48, there is an increase, followed by a decrease at 48 hours or a second "peak." After this point, the levels rise towards 60 hours.

There are basically two peak periods within the 60-hour fasting period illustrated in the chart: the first at 24 hours and a second peak around 48 hours. As this is an approximate gauge used for reference, it should be noted that the levels can vary considerably if you employ low carb eating prior to fasting and/or dry fasting, at least during the first 18-24 hours of an extended fast. The second chart below is a simplified version of the same chart, with similar results, indicating a peak or ideal goal of 24 hours for shifting into autophagy, where the body must search for the old, damaged cellular matter to break down and reuse for building and repairing materials in the production of new cells.

The general direction of achieving autophagy indicates a 24-hour fast as the ideal period for reaching this goal. The peak "dip" indicated in the basic graph above is the peak point that prevails in most charts and diagrams indicating the onset of autophagy.

What happens when we reach the point of autophagy? This is an important step during which our cells shift towards cleaning up the cellular waste and damaged, broken down matter to rebuild. Our bodies have the ability to detect which materials are damaged and will use these first, avoiding already healthy cells and tissues available. When this process begins, at the 24-hour mark, we have several options:

- Continue fasting to continue the benefit the cellular rejuvenation process. As the graphs indicate, this process will continue, on a somewhat consistent level for a period of time, following the first 24 hours

- Break your fast. Autophagy may begin before 24 hours, if your method is dry fasting, and/or if your eating plan includes a significant reduction in carbs and glucose, for at least 24 hours prior to fasting

- Enjoy some bone broth and/or gradually break your fast. This will stop the production of autophagosomes, though it will also infuse a significant amount of nutrients to support your body

Determining when autophagy begins remains vague, with little to no indication of when it begins. Unless we can test our bodies for the presence of autophagosome production, we can only rely on the general guidelines that will lead our bodies to this point, and measure ketones to confirm ketosis as a means to determine that we are close to achieving this goal. Overall, using intermittent fasting along with a low carb or ketogenic diet, is the best way to reach the goal of autophagy and all of its benefits.

Chapter 6: Foods and Nutrients That Support Autophagy and Ketosis

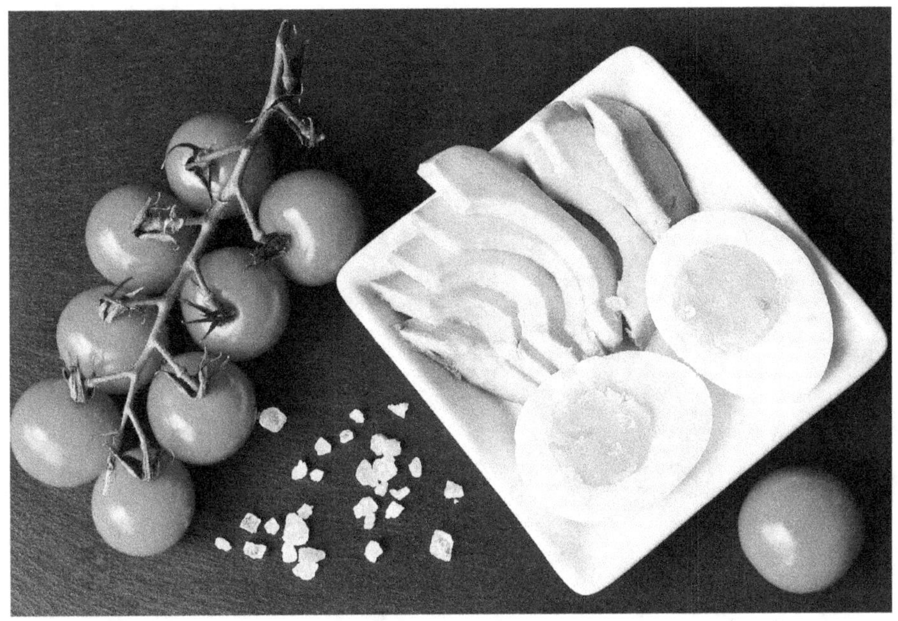

The ketogenic diet is the best way to achieve ketosis while supporting the effectiveness of intermittent fasting to gain amazing benefits of autophagy. Planning meals and funding recipes with low carbs and low glycemic levels doesn't have to be difficult. Most food options are usually available locally and within a reasonable budget. This section focuses on the best options for simple foods that can be used as a foundation to build your diet.

Simple, Key Foods for Ketogenic or Low Carb Diet

Eggs

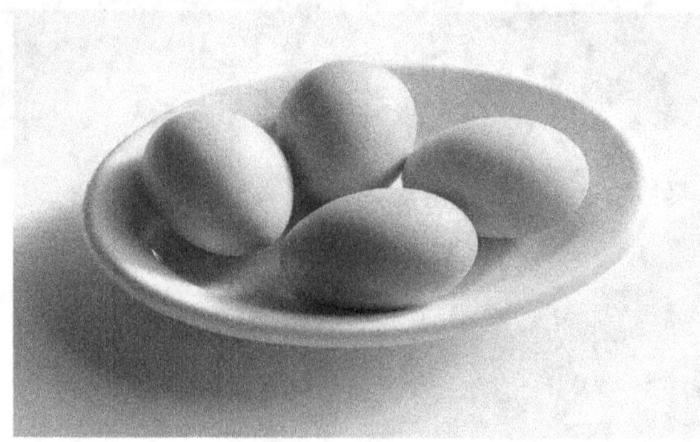

A popular breakfast option, eggs are a good option any time of day within your eating window. They can be prepared in different ways for convenience (boiled or scrambled, for example) and added to almost any meal. On their own, eggs contain enough nutrients to meet some of the daily requirements: omega 3 and 6 fatty acids, protein and calcium are all included in just one serving. Just one or two eggs each day can add a good amount of minerals and fats that your body needs. Eggs are also low in carbohydrates, and glucose, which make them an ideal choice for the ketogenic diet. In baking, eggs are often used and may continue to be included as an ingredient in many recipes, where other items are replaced or modified to accommodate a low carb diet.

Spinach, Kale and Dark Leafy Greens

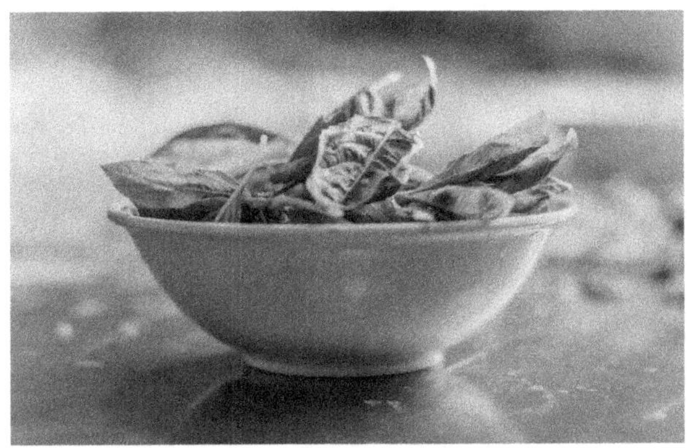

Dark, leafy greens are generally an excellent option because of the rich amount and variety of nutrients they all contain. While there are more dark green leafy options, such as arugula, Swiss chard, and parsley, spinach and kale are often available in most grocery stores and local farmer's markets, which make them easy to include in your diet. Dark greens contain a wealth of vitamins, iron, calcium, and protein. In fact, many vegans and vegetarians can obtain most of their dietary needs from these vegetables. They are most powerful raw when the enzymes remain active, and the nutrients absorbed more thoroughly into the body and used efficiently. These vegetables are also excellent in soups, stir-fries or stews, and can be easily blended into juices and smoothies.

Bone Broth

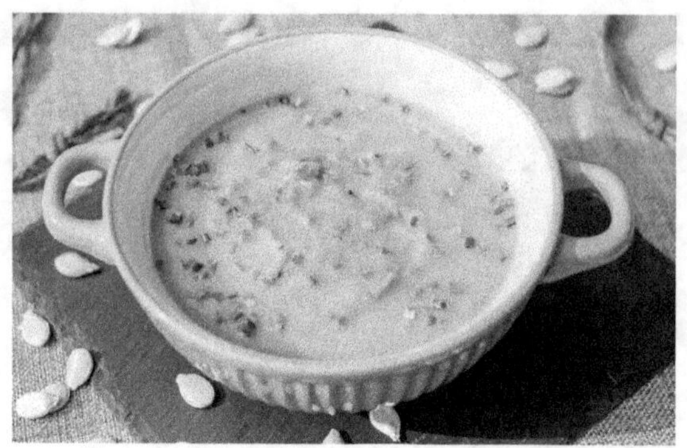

A simple yet very effective way to get most of your nutrients is from bone broth. Chicken and beef are the most common and popular options for these broths. Bone broth can be made from scratch from leftover poultry and beef bones, though the process is time-consuming and can take approximately 24 hours to transfer all of the bones' nutrients into the broth, for maximum nutrition value. For this reason, bone broth can be found in dried powder form for easy preparation, as well as cartons that are ready to heat and serve. Some companies add flavors, such as spices and herbs, to enhance the taste, as broth tends to be very mild and low in flavor. When choosing a broth that is already prepared, be sure to find a good, reputable brand that does not contain preservatives and preferably uses all-natural and organic ingredients.

One of the most important and beneficial ingredients in bone broth is collagen. It is very advantageous to our bone health and provides anti-aging properties as well. Collagen is contained in protein and the main part or component in connective tissue. There are many benefits to taking collagen, whether in bone broth, where is it naturally or in supplement form:

- It reduces joint pain associated with the breakdown of cartilage, as a result of arthritis and similar conditions.
- It is anti-aging in that it promotes better elasticity in skin and tissues
- Reduction in cellulite and toxins stored in the body
- Supports cognitive function and brain health
- Improves digestion and microbial balance (bacterial systems) within the body

If you choose to take collagen as a supplement instead of bone broth, be sure to research the different options available to obtain the most natural, and the best quality available. Bone broth is a convenient and easy way to obtain a lot of nutrients without preparing a complete meal. It's ideal on the go and in between meals. Bone broth can be used during intermittent fasting and as a meal replacement during an eating window if desired.

Berries

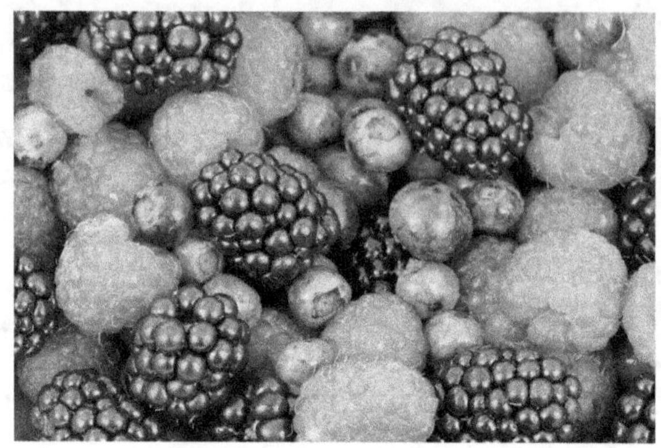

All berries are exceptionally healthy and full of antioxidants, which support the immune system, prevent cancer and other diseases. Strawberries, raspberries, blueberries and blackberries, currants and gooseberries are included in this category, and can be a great snack on their own, served with yogurt or with full fat, sugar-free cream (dairy or non-dairy). Berries are ideal for smoothies and easy to find when in season at local markets and grocery stores. While fresh berries are the best option, some varieties tend to ripen quickly and need to be consumed within a short period of time. For this reason, frozen berries are a good option for smoothies, desserts and can be kept for longer periods of time for convenient use.

Soy

Tofu, tempeh, miso, and soy products, in general, contain most of our daily nutrients and are an ideal replacement for meat and dairy products. While soy is a great way to increase plant-based protein in your diet, it isn't for everyone, particularly people who have allergies or dietary sensitivities related to soy foods. To minimize risks or side effects of soy, which include bloating and occasional issues with digestion, choose organic, high-quality soy products, preferably from a familiar source or company. Fermented soy foods, such as miso and tempeh, contain the protein, calcium, fiber, and vitamins contained in regular soy products, plus B12, which is rarely found in plant-based foods, and usually only in red meats. Vitamin D is usually found in soy products that are fortified to ensure this essential vitamin is included in your diet.

Seafood and Fatty Fish

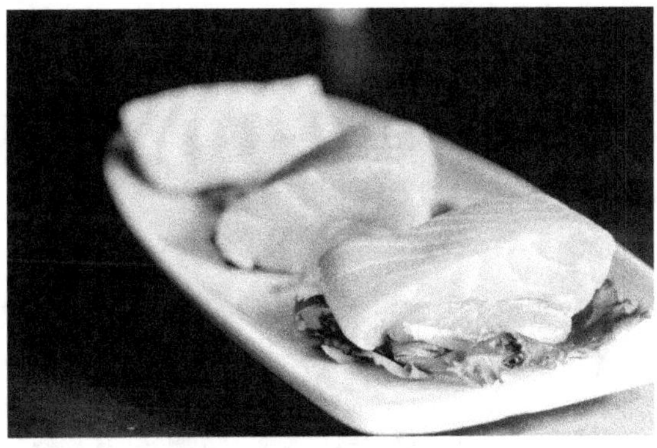

Fish is a good source of healthy fats, protein, and calcium. In a pinch, canned tuna or salmon is a great option to add to a salad or as a side dish. As the main meal, baked or fried fish is a quick way to prepare a dinner or weekend lunch. Even a small portion of fish can be a strong boost to enhance improvements in cognitive function and building muscle. If seafood is not an agreeable option, other meats such as poultry and good quality red meats are good options for increasing iron and protein in your diet.

Sea Vegetables

Kelp and seaweed are examples of sea vegetables that provide a lot of nutrients, such as iron, protein, and various minerals. While they are not always readily available, seaweed has become popular as a snack, in dried sheets, and as a part of sushi cuisine. On its own, seaweed is a good snack option and can be combined with seafood, avocado and/or vegetables for a complete meal.

Avocado

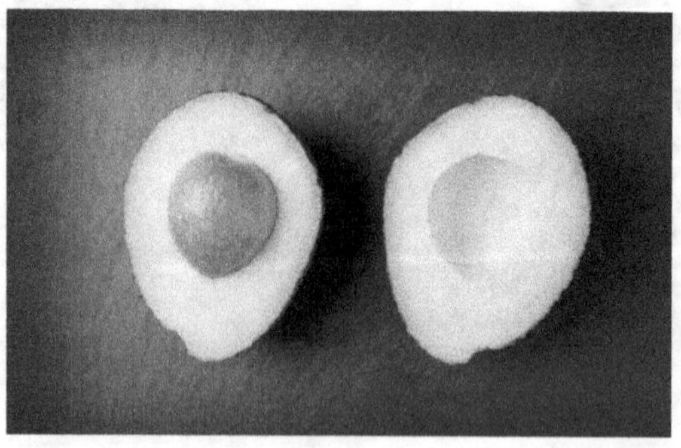

This fruit, which is often mistaken for a vegetable, deserves a category of its own for its numerous benefits. High in fiber, vitamins, and healthy fats, avocado is an ideal food for a low carb or ketogenic diet. It is often considered a superfood because of its high nutrient value. Avocados are filling, and just one serving can complete a meal or snack. They are also excellent as part of a salad, when they are less ripe, or mixed into smoothie, dip or side dish.

Simple Recipes and Meal Suggestions

Scrambled Eggs Skillet

This is a simple, yet effective meal that uses eggs as a base, and adds vegetables, herbs, and other ingredients, as desired, to enhance flavor and add nutrients. An ideal breakfast meal, this dish can be served and enjoyed at any time during your eating window and provides a lot of protein and energy that will last for hours. The ingredients are simple and can be switched and/or replaced, added or omitted as preferred. The recipe below serves 2-3 portions:

- 3-4 eggs (medium or large)
- ½ cup frozen or fresh spinach, sliced in small pieces
- 1 onion, diced into small pieces
- Dried basil, dill, turmeric and/or other spices and/or herbs as desired
- ½ green pepper sliced into small squares, about ½ or

smaller

- 2-3 small mushrooms, sliced thinly
- Sea salt and black pepper (to taste)

Heat a skillet on medium and add 1-2 tablespoons of olive oil. In a small bowl, prepare the eggs by whisking them together, then add to the skillet. Stir and scramble the eggs and reduce the heat. Vegetables included in this recipe can be prepared the night before or just prior to scrambling the eggs so that they are ready to add once the eggs are cooked, or while they are cooking. Add the above ingredients in the following order, to get the most out of their flavor and textures:

- Add spices, salt, and pepper with the eggs in the bowl or while they are scrambled in the skillet
- Herbs can also be added during the scrambling process, or with the vegetables
- Add spinach and green peppers, along with other crunchy or hard-textured vegetables, as they take longer to cook
- Add mushrooms and softer ingredients at the end, as minimal cooking is needed

This dish takes about 10 minutes to cook fully, once all ingredients are in the skillet. The following options may also be considered:

- Diced cubes of ham, smoked salmon, pieces of bacon

(fried or baked prior to the skillet)

- Asparagus is a delicious option, though it takes longer to cook. For best results, steam asparagus in a small or medium pot until gently softened, then add to the skillet.

- Kale can be substituted for spinach, though it has a rougher texture and can take longer to cook. Extra time should be taken into consideration, or fry or steam kale in advance for an easier mix.

Tofu Scramble Skillet

If you are vegan or looking for an alternative to scrambled eggs, the scrambled egg skillet dish above can be made with tofu as the substitute. This option requires a bit more preparation, to add flavor to the tofu by marinating overnight or several hours before this meal is cooked. The best type of tofu to use is extra firm, with little or no additives, or flavors added. This variety of tofu is fairly common and can be found in most grocery stores. The following ingredients are used in the margination process, which is easy to prepare:

- 1 block of extra firm tofu

- 2 cups of vegetable broth (or enough to cover the block of tofu)

- Herbs, spices, and/or flavors to add. This may include the same spices and herbs used in the egg skillet dish.

- Turmeric is recommended for its nutritional value and

pleasant taste. It also adds color to tofu, making it appear more like scrambled eggs.

- Dried bay leaves

Combine all of the ingredients into a medium-sized container that can be sealed and refrigerated. This includes the broth, spices, turmeric, and bay leaves, plus other ingredients as preferred. Pour over the firm tofu or simply add the block to the mixed broth, ensuring there is enough to cover the tofu so that it is fully submerged for marinating. To make it easier, and reduce the amount of broth needed, slice the tofu lengthwise or in large cubes before marinating. The best results of this process require soaking the tofu overnight, though two hours minimum should be sufficient to transfer the bulk of the flavor.

Once the tofu is ready, remove from the fridge and heat the skillet on medium, as you would to scramble eggs. Add olive oil. Drain the broth liquid from the container and retain ¼ or ½ cups to add to the skillet. Mash the tofu in a medium bowl, so that it even, with all pieces of tofu similar in size. Add to the skillet, along with the broth liquid, vegetables and add more spices and herbs as desired.

Options for this dish include adding 1 teaspoon of miso paste to strengthen the flavor. Garlic can also be added.

Shakshuka

Eggs are a feature of this dish, which adds a tomato sauce base, plus herbs and other ingredients. Like the skillet dish, shakshuka can be modified to include or omit ingredients are desired, while retaining the two main ingredients: eggs and tomato sauce. The tomato sauce in this recipe can either be homemade from stewed tomatoes or canned. Canned tomatoes are often the best option for time management, though its best to avoid varieties or brands with added sugars and other preservatives. For this recipe, diced or pureed tomatoes are the best option, as they create a smooth base for poaching eggs. This meal involves just one skillet and can be served directly from the skillet once it is ready or transferred to a deep dish.

To prepare this meal, heat the skillet on medium and add 1-2 tablespoons olive oil. Add the following spices to the oil and reduce to medium-low:

- Sea salt and pepper
- Turmeric
- Chili flakes (optional)
- Basil, oregano
- Cumin (seeds or powder)
- 1 clove crushed garlic

Sautee the above ingredients until they are all coated in oil and soften, which takes about 2-3 minutes. For the next step, add the following:

- 1 cup pureed tomatoes of tomato sauce

- Additional spices and/or herbs, if desired.

Stir the ingredients together, making sure they are all combined evenly, while keeping the cooking level on medium-low, then slightly increasing to medium, add any (all, some or none) of the following:

- Sliced green peppers
- Okra
- Bell peppers
- ½ cup ground beef, chicken or lamb (previously cooked until brown, with added spices)
- Sliced mushrooms

Add more ingredients not included in the list, as required, and continue to cook for another 5-7 minutes. Take two eggs and break them into the mixture, both in a central location of the skillet, so that they can absorb the surrounding flavors as they cook. Adding the two (or three) eggs should be done towards the end of preparing this dish so that they can cook without further stirring or mixing. Once the eggs are cooked and "settled," the dish is ready to serve right from the skillet.

There are many variations to this dish, which include the following toppings and ingredients for consideration:

- Add ½ cup of soft goat cheese or cream cheese to the tomato sauce to create a rose sauce
- Toppings can include dried or fresh parsley, dill,

parmesan cheese or any variety of shredded cheese

- Bacon crumbles, as a topping or mixed into the tomato sauce

Casseroles

<u>Lasagne Options for Low Carb Diets</u>

During the colder seasons, casseroles and similar baking dishes are an excellent and easy way to prepare a meal. From lasagne to moussaka and other blends of vegetables and meats with various sauces and toppings, casseroles provide a hearty meal, and most often, a good portion of leftovers for the next day. A standard oven and a medium to large baking dish are the main requirements for assembling a good casserole meal.

Before you begin to prepare this dish, there are limitless recipes and options available, or you can simply invent your own casserole with the basic foundations of what's involved. This recipe provides a lot of options for changes and substitutes and can be easily adapted to a ketogenic or low carb diet. The first option is to choose the ingredients and "theme" of your casserole:

- Is the base of this dish tomato-based?
- Will cheese be an option as part of the ingredients and/or as a topping?
- Is this meal vegan or vegetarian?

If you choose to add meat to this dish, especially ground beef, pork, lamb and/or chicken, heat a skillet and cook until it is browned and seasoned, then set aside. The portion of meat prepared depends on how large your casserole will be, or simply how much meat you wish to include. This can be anywhere from ½ cup to 2 cups of cooked ground meat. Other ingredients to add may include diced onions, crushed garlic, chili flakes, salt, and pepper.

If you are making a lasagne dish, noodles are traditionally used in the layering process. For a low carb version of this recipe, thinly sliced eggplant, zucchini and/or cabbage leaves all make excellent substitutes. They can be added in between layers of cooked meat, shredded cheese and other vegetables, such as sliced carrots, basil leaves, peppers and/or mushrooms. If zucchini and/or eggplant are used in this recipe, they should be prepared ahead as follows:

- Slice the eggplant and/or zucchini thinly and lengthwise, then rinse in a colander
- Add a thin layer of salt to both sides of each slice and set aside for 20 minutes. This process effectively tenderizes the vegetable, making it easier to bake or cook
- Rinse the salt off the vegetable slices, and pat dry. They are now ready to use in making the lasagne

When preparing a layered casserole dish, including lasagne, always evenly coat the pan with olive oil, then add a thin layer of either tomato sauce or creamy cheese sauce (or a combination of both mixed together). This will keep the bottom of the pan from burning and prevent the ingredients from sticking. Add more layers, beginning with the thinly sliced zucchini and/or eggplant "noodles," or cabbage leaves. The addition or substitution of cabbage leaves will alter the taste of this casserole to a more cabbage-roll flavor, which may be a good option for some occasions. For the cabbage roll-lasagne variation, cheese can be omitted or added as a light topping.

After the initial layer, alternate between different vegetables, and/or meat with a sauce layer in between. In the end or top layer, sprinkle carefully and lightly with olive oil to avoid burning the casserole in the oven. Add a layer of spices, such as paprika, and pepper or sprinkle with shredded cheese or parmesan. Bake in a pre-heated oven for approximately 40 minutes on 350 degrees Fahrenheit. Depending on several factors, such as the number of ingredients, size of the dish, and types of ingredients used, baking may take more or less time. For this reason, check the oven frequently, in 5 to 6-minute intervals, beginning around 25 minutes and after. This will give you a good indication of how quickly the casserole of your choice will take when it is prepared again.

<u>Cauliflower and Broccoli Cheese Bake</u>

If you are looking for a simpler option that requires fewer ingredients and preparation, this option or a variation of this dish is an easy meal. It doesn't require any measurements or specifications, just the desired ingredients and a lot of cheese. If you're are vegan or prefer a plant-based option, there are a vegetable and soy-based vegan cheeses available in most grocery stores. For a creamier option, where the cheese component of this casserole is more rich and thicker, add cream cheese. For best results, melt the cream cheese in a microwave for 30-60 seconds, before adding to the other ingredients.

When you picture a macaroni and cheese bake, this casserole is basically the same idea, with the exception of replacing the noodles with the vegetable(s) of your choice. In combination with cheese flavors, broccoli and cauliflower are excellent options. They contain the right texture and compliment any type of cheese or combination of cheeses. This is also the case for vegan cheese, which tends to taste similar to dairy-based cheese. If it is essential to have vegan cheese that melts similarly to diary cheese, choose vegetable-based cheese options instead of soy-based, which doesn't melt as well.

To prepare this dish, grease a medium or large baking dish with olive oil and preheat the oven to 350 degrees. Prepare the broccoli and cauliflower by removing the stems and chopping the florets into small, 1-inch pieces. If only broccoli or cauliflower are available or only one of these options is preferred, double the amount of your choice. Once the vegetables are chopped equally in size, add to a large bowl and toss in at least 2 cups of shredded cheese, mixing thoroughly to coat. Add or sprinkle the equivalent of 2 teaspoons of olive oil into the bowl. Cheese options (dairy-based) to consider include:

- Shredded mozzarella, cheddar and/or Swiss cheese
- ½ cup of melted cream cheese (plain, unflavoured)

Other ingredients to consider adding to this recipe include:

- Bacon bits or crumble (optional) or the vegan version of the same
- Ground beef or the soy/vegan equivalent, fried or baked in a skillet

Pour the cheese-covered broccoli and/or cauliflower into the casserole dish, and top with paprika, pepper, shredded parmesan cheese and sprinkle with oil. Bake uncovered for 35 minutes. Keep an eye on the top of the casserole, to ensure it doesn't overcook. Additional cheese can be added to the top of this dish halfway through baking if preferred.

If neither cauliflower nor broccoli are available or preferred, brussels sprouts are a great option for baking, especially with parmesan cheese. They can be baked on their own in a medium baking dish, coated in oil and parmesan cheese, until they are slightly crispy on the outside. These make a great side dish or light meal.

Baking Vegetables: Keeping it Simple

There are some vegetables that are simply delicious on their own, with very little or nothing added, as they contain enough flavor on their own to carry a meal or side. The following vegetables are recommended, especially when they are in season and at their peak performance:

- Eggplant. Once prepared by soaking in salt for 20 minutes, eggplant slices can be baked on their own, sprinkled lightly with salt, or coated in parmesan cheese.

- Squash. Any variety of squash is an excellent meal on its own, due to its rich flavor and texture. To prepare, poke holes with a fork into the thick skin of the squash and bake for 10-15 minutes in 350 degrees. This will soften the vegetable and allow easier slicing to further bake for another 30-40 minutes until the inner flesh of the vegetable is tender. Coat with oil or butter before baking.

- Potatoes, yams, and sweet potatoes. All of these options take a while to bake, at least one hour, which makes them best to prepare when you have time to spare, or while preparing another dish. Smaller sizes of this vegetable bake faster. For good results, wrap in tin foil and poke with a fork to allow more even cooking.

- Radishes. This pungent tasting vegetable becomes much milder once it is roasted in the oven for 15-20 minutes. It can be cooked similarly to brussels sprouts, only without any added ingredients, with the exception of salt, butter or oil.

- Turnip or Rutabaga. This root vegetable becomes milder in flavor once it is baked. It is also used as a low carb alternative to potatoes and/or yams. These root vegetables can be shredded and fried similarly to potatoes or baked as well.

In general, root vegetables make great baking dishes, on their own or with other foods. Salt and olive oil or butter are the only ingredients needed to enhance the flavors of baked vegetables. They can also be baked in a small, covered baking dish with oil, salt and pepper and broth to add more flavor if desired. Miso paste can be added for more nutrients.

Salads

There are many options for salads, as there are ingredients to consider. Salads are a great opportunity to get the most out of leafy green vegetables while adding many other flavors to sweeten, spice or otherwise liven up the bitter flavors of arugula, spinach, and kale. Lettuce is another good option for a salad base, as it is neutral in flavor and offers a good source of iron and fiber. Kale, spinach, arugula and/or Swiss chard all offer a high level of nutrients and can be used either in combination or individually as a salad base. To build a salad, there are a few items to consider before preparation:

- Choose your base, preferably a leafy green: kale, cabbage, spinach, arugula, swiss chard, lettuce and/or others. Slice the green thin and combine in a large bowl

- Add to your greens: sprouts (pea sprouts, alfalfa, bean sprouts, etc.), other vegetables, such as carrots, broccoli, cucumber, edamame beans (shelled)

The dressing doesn't need to be fancy or loaded with ingredients. A simple balsamic dressing with oil and vinegar is healthy, low in carbohydrates and sugar, and very easy to make within a few minutes:

- Create a balsamic dressing by combining vinegar, olive oil (about 2-3 tablespoons each), and add flavor: freshly squeezed lime or lemon juice, dried rosemary leaves (crushed), mashed raspberries, or another option

Once the base ingredients are combined, and dressing is prepared, there are many toppings and other ingredients to consider adding to mix or on top of the salad:

- Baked chicken breast in basil leaves and olive oil (sliced into strips as a topping)
- Baked salmon
- Fried shrimp with butter and garlic
- Spicy tofu or tempeh cubes
- Shredded cheese (any variety)
- Nuts and seeds (pumpkin, flax or hemp seeds; almonds, walnuts, peanuts, cashews, hazelnuts, etc.). Nuts can be

added raw, lightly salted or dry roasted on the stovetop, before adding as a topping to a salad

- Roasted root vegetables, such as baked squash or yams, sliced into cubes. Roasted or pickled beets are another option
- Boiled egg

There are countless ways to change and dress a salad, either for a regular meal or as a side dish. Salads that focus primarily on nutrient-rich and low carb ingredients are ideal before an intermittent fasting window or long-term fast. Salads are also a gentle way to effectively break a fast, as they provide a lot of healthy ingredients while not overwhelming the digestive system right after fasting.

Soups and Stews

A slow-cooked meal is a tasty option, though often overlooked in a busy society where meals are prepared quickly and without much thought. Soups and stews are best made over a period of hours, which can be done with a slow cooker while you're away at work, or overnight in preparation for the next day. Making large portions is advantageous for meal preparation over a week or several days in advance. Preparing a stew is as easy as choosing a broth or soup base, herbs, and spices, as well as the ingredients. Beef stew is an exceptional way to add a significant source of iron, protein, and calcium to a meal, along with other vegetables and spices to add fiber and vitamins, including antioxidants. Meat can be substituted for tempeh or tofu, and a vegetable soup base or broth can be flavored further with miso or soy sauce.

The broth or soup base should be as natural as possible, either through careful selection at a grocery store or by preparing the broth homemade with soup bones and vegetable rinds. The broth or base should be plain, and all spices and flavors added, such as bay leaves, sea salt, pepper, basil and other options as desired. Turmeric and paprika make great options as well.

Stewing beef should be added first to the broth, as it takes the longest to cook. Other vegetables and ingredients can be added later, once the beef is cooked and becomes tender:

- Celery (sliced in small, bite-sized pieces)
- Carrots, sliced
- Potatoes cut into cubes (or turnips, for a low carb option)
- Asparagus
- Spinach
- Onion (minced)
- Garlic cloves (crushed)
- Chili flakes and/or cayenne pepper

Soy sauce can be added in small amounts to boost the flavor of the stew. Salt and pepper are also good options to enhance the beef flavor. Stewing this dish can be easily done over a period of

6-8 hours on low heat. The recommended amount of broth or soup base is eight cups or more, to ensure all of the ingredients are covered and submerged. Adding more ingredients and using a larger cooking pot would require more broth.

Soup Options

Creamy soups are often coconut milk or dairy milk-based and can add another level of taste to a simple soup. Curried soups are usually prepared with a coconut milk base, with spices including curry powder, added. Preparing a curry soup is as simple as adding coconut milk and curry spices to a vegetable or meat-based broth or soup base, then adding the ingredients. To make a soup creamy, simply add cream to the broth, along with the various vegetables. Once the ingredients are cooked, remove from the heat and blend in a food processor, then reheat to serve.

If you are looking to add healthy, natural sources of carbs for energy to a soup, consider lentils, chickpeas, kidney beans, and black beans as options, as well as barley and quinoa as healthy grain options that also provide a high nutrient count. Avoid refined pasta and rice as much as possible and add as many whole food options. Ideal vegetables to blend for creamy or thickening soups include pumpkin (in pureed form), squash and carrots. Broccoli, potato, and cauliflower are options that may be added together or separately to make a hearty soup.

Chili Options

Like stews, chilis are a great way to provide a filling meal, while staying warm during colder months. Chili is traditionally made with beans, though this option can be omitted to adjust for a lower carb version. Tomato paste and sauce are the first ingredients to begin with, which can be made at home or store-bought. Stewing tomatoes with pureed sauce and paste can be further enhanced with sliced tomatoes, so that they can be stewed to absorb the flavors, in combination with cayenne, chili flakes, black pepper, and paprika. Ground beef or a vegetarian meat substitute is added to stir with the tomato sauce, followed by the following ingredients:

- Sliced green peppers and/or bell peppers
- Diced jalapeno peppers (sliced thinly)
- Okra
- Zucchini (sliced)
- Mushrooms
- Spinach
- Onions (diced)
- Garlic (crushed)

Chili is stewed slowly, over a period of a few hours, to get the most flavor out of all ingredients combined. The longer the duration, the stronger the flavor. If a large enough stew is prepared, the chili can last for several days as a main meal or in combination with other foods. It makes a great dinner or small portion size with eggs in the morning. As a light meal, it can be served in a bowl topped with shredded cheese or with salad.

Smoothies

One of the best ways to get nutrients quickly and efficiently is with a smoothie or milkshake. If you have any variety of milk (dairy or non-dairy), various fruits and some ice in the freezer, you already have most, if not all the basic ingredients to make a smoothie. In addition to the basics, there are other options to add for boost the protein and nutrient levels in your smoothie, including:

- Any variety of nut butter, such as peanut, almond, hazelnut or sesame butter. Just one tablespoon can provide a substantial amount of protein in your smoothie

- Most smoothies add a banana for its thickening effect and the added flavor. Avocados make a great low carb alternative to bananas and can be added to almost any combination of fruits. On their own, avocados are a great milkshake combined with coconut, almond or dairy milk as a base.

- Hemp seeds, flax seeds, and plant-based proteins: these can be either crushed into a powder or small granules, like hemp or flax or bought as a fine powder in most bulk stores. The types of plant-based proteins are limitless and include everything from soy, pumpkin, hemp and chia seed varieties. Chia seeds on their own make another great addition, due to their high calcium and fiber.

- MCT oil or coconut oil. This is a beneficial way to add more healthy fats to your diet, especially if you adhere to a strict ketogenic diet. MCT oil is not as common in grocery stores as coconut oil, though it can be ordered online or purchased in most natural food stores.

- Kale, spinach and other leafy greens can make an excellent addition to a fruit-based smoothie. Their strong, bitter flavor is offset by the natural sweetness of watermelon, cantaloupe, and other melon juices, or mango and orange juice. If you choose to use juice as a base instead of milk, avoid the packaged variety and try making your own homemade juice with a juicer, blender or by simply hand-squeezing citrus fruits. Watermelon is a good choice, due to how quickly it can be blended in a food processor and added to a smoothie. Mangoes and citrus fruits combined also make a great option as a base for a green smoothie

- Green tea, more specifically matcha, is usually available in powder form and makes a great energy boost to any smoothie. There is a high level of antioxidants in green tea that rival many fresh fruits and vegetables. If fresh or frozen fruits are limited, green tea powder is a good substitute with coconut milk and either avocado or banana.

New supplements, "boosters" and various nutrient enhancements are becoming more readily available, with more plant-based and low carb options that include high levels of vitamins, proteins, and ingredients not always available in fresh fruits and vegetables. These are especially beneficial for long-term shelf life and increasing the meal replacement value of a smoothie, which can be a great option for breakfast or in between meals as a snack. The following ingredient combinations are suggestions for different flavors, and can be modified or changed according to personal preference:

<u>Low Carb Smoothie Options:</u>

- Avocado (ripe), coconut milk, matcha green tea powder and low carb sweetener (monk fruit or stevia)
- Berries, almond milk (or dairy, coconut milk) with tahini (sesame butter)
- Dark cocoa (unsweetened) with almond milk, peanut or hazelnut butter
- Pumpkin puree, cinnamon and almond milk with hemp seeds or protein powder

<u>Moderate Carb/High Energy Options for Workouts:</u>

- Bananas, avocado, coconut or almond milk, and low carb sweetener

- Berries, bananas, milk, and hemp protein

- Mangoes, coconut milk, cardamom powder and low carb sweetener (peaches can also be used as a substitute)

<u>Juice-Based Smoothies:</u>

- Orange juice, mangoes, bananas, and pumpkin protein powder

- Watermelon (or cantaloupe, honeydew) with pineapple, mango and/or peaches. Add lime or lime and leafy greens, such as kale, mint or spinach leaves

Another option to consider adding to a smoothie for flavor, nutrients, and thickening the texture is yogurt or kefir. Both options contain bacterial cultures beneficial for gut health and are best used in a plain, unsweetened form. Kefir contains a higher level of probiotics and tends to be thinner than regular yogurt, which makes it an ideal option for smoothies. Yogurt, while it is thicker, can be added to almond or coconut milk. Yogurt and kefir-based smoothies can be prepared similarly to milk and non-dairy milk-based varieties.

Fermented Foods

One of the healthiest types of foods on the planet is fermented vegetables, dairy, and soy. The most familiar varieties are yogurt and kefir for dairy, tempeh, and miso for soy and kimchi and sauerkraut for vegetables. All fermented foods have a direct impact on improving gut health, which is essential in digesting and properly utilizing all of the nutrients we receive from the foods we eat. Fermented foods are also very convenient and often available in most grocery stores or delis. They have been associated with the prevention of certain cancers, and digestive diseases, and promote weight loss while supporting the metabolism. The strong level of nutrients in kimchi and sauerkraut make them ideal side dishes, which is usually how they are served, either on the side of a dish or in a small bowl. These foods are also very filling in small doses and can be used sparingly with stews and stir fry meals.

Sauerkraut, kimchi, and yogurt can be made at home by following a recipe or bought already prepared for convenience. Fermented soy, such as miso and tempeh, go through a longer process. In order to produce miso, the fermentation process can take weeks, months, and for some varieties, years to make. The longer the duration of fermenting, the stronger the taste and flavor. Miso is beneficial in small amounts in soups, dips and as an added ingredient to stews and sautés. Fermented foods have a long shelf life and once opened, can be refrigerated for at least one week or more.

All of the above foods, recipes, suggestions, and ideas can build a solid start to a healthy diet that can support intermittent fasting and prepare the body for longer-term fasting goals.

Overall, most people don't always take into consideration the quality of foods they eat when they consider fasting as an option, and instead, focus on the fasting process itself. While this is important, the foods we eat around those fasting windows is equally vital to ensuring we have all the nutrients we require to sustain our bodies through a fast, and as we move towards a state of autophagy.

Chia Seed Puddings

A simple yet very effective way to increase the nutrient content of your meal is by adding chia seeds. They contain a significant source of plant-based protein, calcium, vitamins, fiber, and antioxidants. Chia seeds are great for creating puddings from milk, as they expand in liquid and create a thick, custard-like texture. Their taste adapts to the ingredients combined with them, and they are excellent for vegan diets that are also low carb or ketogenic. In its simple form, chia seed pudding can be prepared as follows:

- 2 cups milk (dairy, coconut or almond milk)
- ½ cup full-fat cream (dairy or coconut cream)
- 2-3 teaspoons low carb sweetener (monk fruit, stevia or a blend)
- 1 teaspoon vanilla extract

Combine all of the ingredients in a medium to large bowl and mix evenly, to ensure all chia seeds are distributed throughout the milk. Add cinnamon and more sweetener as needed. Refrigerate for at least two hours to thicken the pudding and serve. Preparing this dish and refrigerating overnight is a good option for enjoying immediately in the morning, with no further preparation time needed. There are many other flavors and options to consider when preparing this pudding by adding the following:

- Sprinkle the top of the pudding with cinnamon or cardamom just prior to serving
- Combine fresh fruits, such as berries and currents, to enhance the flavor of the pudding. These can be added during the mixing of the ingredients, or later, once the pudding has formed.
- Add dark cocoa or chocolate (unsweetened) to the pudding, along with chocolate flakes or shavings as a topping or ingredient.
- Coconut flakes, slivered almonds, crushed pecans, walnuts or pistachios are all great options to add flavor to the pudding
- Hemp hearts and flax seeds can enhance the healthy fats and protein content of the pudding.

Chia seed pudding offers a lot of options to mix and match various flavors and experiment with your own tastes. The best advantage of this dish is its dessert-like quality, which is also very nutritious and fitting as a full meal in itself. It can serve as a meal replacement at any time of day.

How Does Intermittent Fasting Combine with a Low Carb Diet?

Implementing both a fasting schedule with dietary changes is an involving task, though it provides a lot of options on planning and scheduling. The following sample plans indicate how to use various diet options in conjunction with intermittent fasting plans, starting from 12:12 (twelve hours fasting, twelve hours eating) as a starting point:

12:12 Intermittent Fasting Sample: Plan A

This plan begins the beginner level of fasting for 12 hours at an early 6 am start.

12:12 sample daily plan (any weekday or weekend)	Fasting/eating schedule from 6 am to 6 pm
6 am	Begin eating window. Coffee or tea, water. Scrambled eggs or tofu with fresh fruit or avocado
12 pm – 1 pm	Lunch break: salad with baked salmon and a side of kimchi
3 pm	Snack (optional). Yogurt with fruit, or a smoothie

| 5 pm – 6 pm | Dinner: baked casserole or stew with a side salad
Coffee or tea |
| 6 pm until 6 am the following day | Fasting begins immediately after dinner and lasts for 12 hours until the following day at 6 am when breakfast is served. |

12:12 Intermittent Fasting Sample: Plan B

This version or option for the 12-hour fasting plan begins slightly later in the morning, at 8am. This can be further shifted to begin at 9, or 10 am, though keep in mind the duration of the eating window ends exactly 12 hours later, into the late evening:

12:12 sample daily plan (any weekday or weekend)	Fasting/eating schedule from 8 am to 8 pm
8 am	Begin eating window. Coffee or tea, water. Scrambled eggs or tofu with fresh fruit or avocado
1 pm – 2 pm	Lunch break: salad with baked salmon and a side of kimchi
4 pm	Snack (optional). Yogurt with fruit, or a smoothie
6 pm – 8 pm	Dinner: baked casserole or stew with a side salad Coffee or tea
8 pm until 8 am	Fasting begins immediately after dinner

the following day	and lasts for 12 hours until the following day at 6 am when breakfast is served.

16:8 Intermittent Fasting Sample: Plan A

After a few weeks of 12:12, moving into a longer fasting phase is recommended to adjust your body to a longer period of abstaining from food and drink. The following sample uses the same food options as 12:12 to illustrate how they would be adjusted to accommodate a change in hours. The significant change is in the increase of 12 to 16 hours of fasting while maintaining a similar eating schedule:

16:8 sample daily plan (any weekday or weekend)	Fasting/eating schedule from 6 am to 2 pm
6 am	Begin eating window. Coffee or tea, water. Scrambled eggs or tofu with fresh fruit or avocado.
11 am – 12 pm	Lunch break: salad with baked salmon and a side of kimchi. A mid-morning snack is also an option, such as yogurt with chia seeds and fruits or a smoothie.
1 pm - 2 pm	Light lunch or mid-afternoon snack. The two eating options suggested between 11 am – 12 pm and 1 – 2 pm can be interchangeable, depending on your

	schedule and preference.
2 pm – 6 am the next morning	Fasting begins at 2 pm and lasts until the next day at 6 am. Dinner is skipped completely. Bone broth and/or tea are options during the fasting period.

<u>16:8 Intermittent Fasting Sample: Plan B</u>

The following sample starts at a later time to show how traditional meals can be further adjusted within the 8-hour range. In plan A, the dinner is skipped completely, with a focus on breakfast and lunch, with an option for a mid-morning or mid-afternoon snack. In this schedule, the eating window begins later, after breakfast:

16:8 sample daily plan (any weekday or weekend)	**Fasting/eating schedule from 10 am to 6 pm**
10 am	Begin eating window. Smoothie with fruit and protein or yogurt, chia seeds and fresh fruits. Prior to 10 am, during a fasting window, bone broth, coffee, and tea are options.
1 pm – 2 pm	Lunch break: salad with baked salmon and a side of kimchi. This lunch period can be shifted to a later start time, between 2-3 pm.
5 pm – 6 pm	Dinner options include a casserole, stir fry

	or skillet meal or baked vegetables with a choice of protein.
6 pm – 10 am the next morning	Fasting begins at 6 pm and lasts until the next day at 10 am. Breakfast is either skipped the next morning completely or moved to a later time, starting 10 am or later. Bone broth and/or tea are options during the fasting period.

16:8 Intermittent Fasting Sample: Plan C:

Applying the same 8-hour fasting window as in plans A and B for the 16:8 fasting schedule, the following option is ideal for late shift work or a later start in the day:

16:8 sample daily plan (any weekday or weekend)	Fasting/eating schedule from 1 pm to 9 pm
1 pm	Begin the eating window and break your fast with a light salad, followed by a nutritious lunch: stir fry, lasagne, soup or stew. Sushi with a side of edamame beans and/or kimchi.
5 pm – 7 pm	Dinner can be served at this time. This may include a skillet, soup, stew or chili. No further meals are required following the dinner, or a light snack can be added

	just prior to beginning the fasting window.
8 pm – 9 pm	A light snack is optional and may include fresh fruits, black olives with guacamole and/or cheese or miso soup with tofu and seaweed.
9 pm – 1 pm the next day	Fasting begins at 9 pm and lasts until the next day at 1 pm. Breakfast is skipped completely, and a light snack or meal can be enjoyed as lunch. Bone broth and/or tea are options during the fasting period.

The next step in the progression to longer fasting intervals is a slight increase from 16 to 18 hours of fasting. While this may not seem like a significant change, the two-hour difference can signify the start of autophagy, which can begin as early as 18 hours into a fasting window. For most people, this process doesn't begin until 24 hours, though there is a chance that some of the benefits could start as early as 18 hours, which makes this step all the more crucial in adapting to this diet.

<u>18:6 Intermittent Fasting Sample: Plan A:</u>

The 18:6 intermittent fasting schedule allows for a 6-hour window for eating, which represents one-quarter of a full 24-hour day. To get the most out of this plan, center your eating plan around two meals instead of three, and include as many nutrients as possible. The sample meals below are simply guidelines, which can be replaced with other options:

18:6 sample daily plan (any weekday or weekend)	Fasting/eating schedule from 7 am to 1 pm

7 am	Begin the eating window with a hearty breakfast, which may include eggs, tofu, fresh herbs, skillet-fried vegetables with a side of bacon or ham and a small bowl of fruit. This meal essentially breaks the fast from the night before, which lasts from 1 pm to 7 am.
10:30 am – 11 am	Lunch can be served at an earlier time, between 10:30 and 1 pm, or this small timeframe can be a suitable option for a mid-morning snack, followed by lunch or larger meal between 12 pm – 1 pm.
12 pm – 1 pm	This is the last meal prior to beginning the fasting window. Add as many nutrients and proteins as possible. If you plan to eat a spicy meal, add a small cup of yogurt to aid in digestion. This is a good option for any dish, particularly where foods can be challenging or slow to digest, such as certain spices and meats.
1 pm – 7 am the next morning	Fasting begins at 1 pm and lasts until the next day at 7 am. Dinner is skipped completely. Bone broth and/or tea are options during the fasting period.

18:6 Intermittent Fasting Sample: Plan B:

The second 18:6 option or plan starts the eating window later in the morning, omitting breakfast completely and focusing on lunch and an early dinner. To get the most out of this plan, center your eating around the lunch hour, adding an optional light snack before and/or after and include as many nutrients as possible. The sample meals below are simply guidelines, which can be replaced with other options:

18:6 sample daily plan (any weekday or weekend)	Fasting/eating schedule from 11 am to 5 pm
11 am	Begin the eating window with a light mid-morning snack, such as avocado, one or two boiled eggs, and miso soup. A chia seed pudding and/or yogurt with fruits are good options. This meal essentially breaks the fast from the night before, which lasts from 5 pm to 11 am.
1 pm – 2 pm	Lunch can be served at an earlier time, between 1 pm and 2 pm, followed by dinner or a larger meal between 4 pm – 5 pm.
4 pm – 5 pm	This is the last meal prior to beginning the fasting window. Add as many nutrients and proteins as possible. If you plan to eat

	a spicy meal, add a small cup of yogurt to aid in digestion. This is a good option for any dish, particularly where foods can be challenging or slow to digest, such as certain spices and meats.
5 pm – 11 am the next morning	Fasting begins at 5 pm and lasts until the next day at 11 am. Breakfast is skipped completely. Bone broth and/or tea are options during the fasting period.

The final suggested plan starts at lunch and allows for more flexibility between the lunch and dinner meals while skipping breakfast entirely. For added nutrients in the morning, enjoy a cup of bone broth and coffee. Drink plenty of water during the fasting hours.

18:6 Intermittent Fasting Sample: Plan C:

18:6 sample daily plan (any weekday or weekend)	Fasting/eating schedule from 1 pm to 7 pm
1 pm	Begin the eating window with a light salad or snack, followed by a lunch that contains a lot of nutrients. This meal essentially breaks the fast from the night before, which lasts from 7 pm to 1 pm
4 pm – 5 pm	Dinner can be served at an earlier time,

	preferably between 4 pm – 5 pm. A light snack may also be added around 3 pm as an appetizer, or as a more substantial snack or dessert after this meal.
6 pm – 7 pm	This is the last meal prior to beginning the fasting window. Even a small portion snack or light meal can contain a lot of nutrients. If you plan to eat a spicy meal, add a small cup of yogurt to aid in digestion. This is a good option for any dish, particularly where foods can be challenging or slow to digest, such as certain spices and meats.
7 pm – 1 pm the next day	Fasting begins at 7 pm and lasts until the next day at 1 pm Breakfast is skipped completely. Bone broth and/or tea are options during the fasting period.

The next phase in intermittent fasting is moving from 18 hours to 20 hours, bringing the "sweet spot" or peak of autophagy even closer. 20 hours marks an important milestone, as it is usually the last stop before trying a full day 24-hour fast. The 20:4 method focuses mostly on one meal or series of healthy foods within a 4-hour window of opportunity:

20:4 Intermittent Fasting Sample: Plan A

20:4 sample daily plan (any weekday or weekend)	Fasting/eating schedule from 8 am to 12 pm
8 am to 12 pm	This is a four-hour fasting window that can begin with either a light start, such as a bowl of fresh fruit and cream, or yogurt, followed by an egg dish loaded with as many nutrients and vitamins as possible. If you start work or become busy within this eating window, be sure to add another small meal or snack within the 11 am to 12 pm or final hour of the window, just prior to beginning the fast.
12 pm – 8 am	Fasting begins at 12 pm, following a light lunch or healthy snack, and lasts until 8 am the next morning. Drink plenty of water, and supplement with bone broth or tea if needed. Coffee can also be added during this time. To increase the chances of achieving autophagy during a 20-hour fast, try dry fasting by omitting all fluids during the fasting window. This will allow your body to use up its resources faster.

Using the same meal ideas in the first plan, the 4-hour window can be moved to a later time in the day, to focus around lunch hour. This is particularly useful is you have a flexible schedule that will accommodate a snack during a break and lunch. Breakfast and dinner meals are omitted completely:

<u>20:4 Intermittent Fasting Sample: Plan B</u>

20:4 sample daily plan (any weekday or weekend)	Fasting/eating schedule from 11 am to 3 pm
11 am to 3 pm	This is a four-hour fasting window that can begin with either a light start, such as a bowl of fresh fruit and cream, or yogurt, followed by an egg dish loaded with as many nutrients and vitamins as possible. This meal can either serve as a late breakfast or early lunch. If you start work or become busy within this eating window, be sure to add another small meal or snack within the 2 pm to 3 pm or final hour of the window, just prior to beginning the fast.
3 pm – 11 am	Fasting begins at 3 pm, following a light lunch or healthy snack, and lasts until 8 am the next morning. Drink plenty of

	water, and supplement with bone broth or tea if needed. Coffee can also be added during this time. To increase the chances of achieving autophagy during a 20-hour fast, try dry fasting by omitting all fluids during the fasting window. This will allow your body to use up its resources faster.

The following two samples plans C and D, illustrate the increased flexibility of a reduced eating window, and the availability to move the preferred mealtimes within those hours. As restrictive as the time frame may appear, the plan itself allows for variances in when the hours are scheduled and can provide opportunities to learn and discover which time of the day works best for eating versus fasting:

20:4 Intermittent Fasting Sample: Plan C

20:4 sample daily plan (any weekday or weekend)	Fasting/eating schedule from 6 am to 10 am
6 am to 10 am	This is a four-hour fasting window that can begin with either a light start, such as a bowl of fresh fruit and cream, or yogurt, followed by an egg dish loaded with as

	many nutrients and vitamins as possible. If you start work or become busy within this eating window, be sure to add another small meal or snack within the 9 am, and 10 am or final hour of the window, just prior to beginning the fast. This specific plan works within the breakfast hours of the day, which can have the benefit of spreading out two meals or light snacking throughout this time frame until fasting begins at 10 am.
10 am – 6 am	Fasting begins at 10 am, following a light lunch or healthy snack, and lasts until 6 am the next morning. Drink plenty of water, and supplement with bone broth or tea if needed. Coffee can also be added during this time. Lunch and dinner are skipped in favor of maximizing the nutrients and good food choices within the early hours of the day. To increase the chances of achieving autophagy during a 20-hour fast, try dry fasting by omitting all fluids during the fasting window. This will allow your body to use up its resources faster.

<u>20:4 Intermittent Fasting Sample: Plan D</u>

20:4 sample daily plan (any weekday or weekend)	Fasting/eating schedule from 4 pm to 8 pm
4 pm to 8 pm	This is a four-hour fasting window that can begin with a salad or soup, followed by a casserole, skillet meal, or similar dish. As the evening progresses, there is the option for a light snack, such as yogurt, fresh fruit, or an egg or avocado, prior to beginning the fasting window at 8 pm. If you have a tendency to become hungry in the morning, be sure to include a lot of nutritious, slow-digesting foods. Include fermented food options within the 4-hour window, and this will help the next morning. This specific plan works around the dinner hour, which can have the benefit of spreading out two meals or light snacking throughout this time frame until fasting begins at 8 pm.
8 pm to 4 pm the	Fasting begins at 8 pm. Drink plenty of

next day	water, and supplement with bone broth or tea if needed. Coffee can also be added during this time.
	Breakfast and lunch are skipped in favor of maximizing the nutrients and good food choices within the evening hours of the day.
	To increase the chances of achieving autophagy during a 20-hour fast, try dry fasting by omitting all fluids during the fasting window. This will allow your body to use up its resources faster.

The 24-hour fasting method is your ideal goal to reach autophagy and moving through all of the shorter intermittent fasting plans will place you in a position for success. As you approach this as your next option, keep the following in mind as you prepare to begin a full day fast:

- Start your first 24-hour fast with plenty of water and acceptable liquids. Avoid dry fasting unless you have tried shorter fasting periods with no fluids or have completed a regular full-day fast several times successfully.

- Prior to ending your eating window, eat a hearty, nutritious meal within the last hour before you begin your fast. This will give your body a good foundation for using high-quality nutrients right up until the process of autophagy begins

- Exercise during the early part of your fast, to increase the metabolic rate, which can move you into autophagy faster as well.

- Bone broth is a good option to keep the nutrient level high during your fast, though it may have the effect of slowing down progression towards autophagy. If you are able to avoid most fluids, and only use water during the fast, this is an ideal situation. Water fasting ensures that you don't lose any hydration during the fasting process.

- Take time to meditate and slowly ease yourself into the fasting window. Don't view this process as a shift from one extreme to another, but rather as a transition from using food to taking a break during the fasting window. Your body will adjust, even if the initial experiences are challenging and with feelings of hunger. These symptoms will pass over time and make your body stronger and more resilient.

- Keep your schedule the same, if possible, and make sure you are getting enough hours of sleep. If you are content with the level of sleep and activities in your life currently, avoid making any radical or significant changes, as this will only cause more stress during the intermittent fasting process. The idea is to make this process as easy and gentle as possible.

As with longer fasting periods, which last over 24 hours, the same principles apply to the preparation and getting used to the new benefits and long-term opportunities that fasting and autophagy have to offer.

Chapter 7: Different Goals and Reasons for Using Autophagy and Low Carb Eating in Life

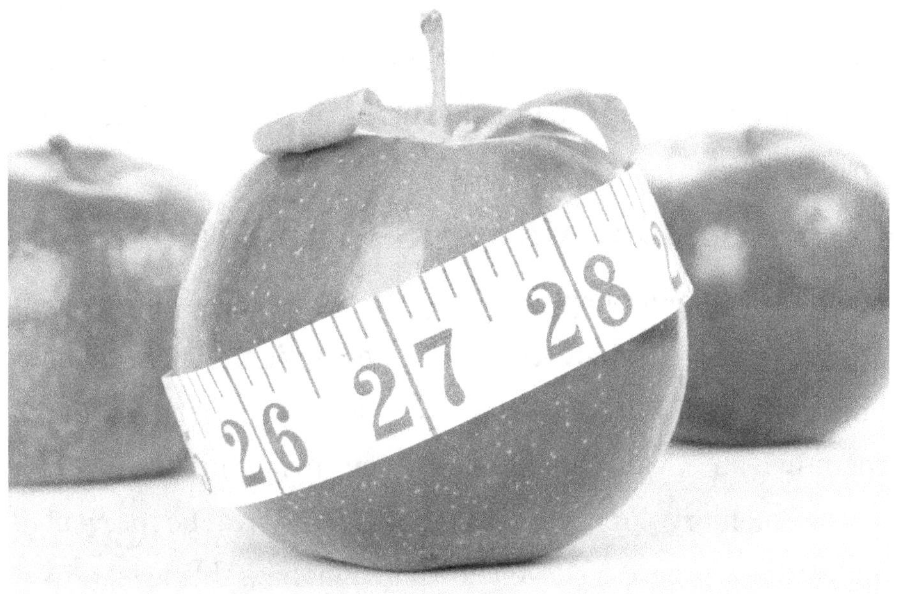

Disease Prevention

Autophagy is one of the best defenses against disease prevention because it functions so effectively at the cellular level. In maximizing the quality production of healthy cells, the chances of mutated and damaged cell production, often resulting from free radicals and other toxins in the body, are minimized, because of the food we eat and the opportunity we give our bodies to reuse the cell and tissue waste that would otherwise cause more problems in our bodies, if left as is.

Examples of the types of diseases and conditions that can be prevented or treated during autophagy include lowering cholesterol and maintaining healthy blood pressure level, preventing Alzheimer's and inflammation in the brain and body, and improving the function of the intestines and digestive system.

Cognitive Function and Brain Health

The nature of autophagy is to improve the quality and function of our body through cellular regeneration. This includes improving the way our brain functions, including memory, cognitive abilities, and focus. In improving how our brain works, memory loss and related diseases can be prevented and/or their progress slowed down to a manageable level.

Weight Loss

One of the most popular reasons to strive for ketosis and autophagy is the benefits of weight loss. Burning fat for fuel instead of glucose is a direct way of losing weight while increasing energy levels and other advantages that follow. There are many case studies that indicate how easily the body can move into a fat-adapted state and continuously burn for weeks or months at a time, while ketosis is regularly achieved.

Treatment of disease and disorders

While autophagy continues to be researched and studied to document its effects, some of the key findings to date include the prevention and treatment of some common diseases. One of the fascinating aspects of this process is the ability to suppress and reverse certain cancerous growths, including tumors. While the cellular regeneration process breaks down old cell waste for repairing damaged tissue and building new cells, it may also inhibit cancerous or mutated cell growth, either stopping or slowing the progression in its tracks. The very nature of autophagy is to promote and strengthen the growth of new cells, so that they perform and function better than before, preventing the start of many diseases of conditions.

The rebuilding and strengthening process at a cellular level would support an improved defense against certain heart conditions and their progression. Certain autoimmune and chronic conditions, such as arthritis, fibromyalgia, as well as inflammation and diseases that impact digestion may also improve over time due to autophagy.

Strengthening the Immune System

Stronger, newer cells will build a solid foundation for an immune system that functions well and can fight off viruses and disease more effectively. While our dietary habits play a key role in building and maintaining and supporting a powerful immune system, the recycling effect of old cells to produce more efficient cellular material can impact every aspect of the way our body functions, from prevention to treatment of mild to serious conditions. If your health is generally good and there are no known conditions, autophagy will continue to keep your immunity level at a high functioning rate, even as we age.

Anti-aging: The Ultimate Benefit of Autophagy

As popular as weight loss is for diet and fasting, as well as the benefits of treating disease, one major fascination with the science of autophagy is its ability to slow down, and to some degree, possibly reverse the aging process. As cells regenerate in smaller numbers as we age, their quality becomes increasingly more important. Some studies indicate that these newer cells have a restorative effect on our bodies, and organs, resulting in improved function. Visually, the skin may become firmer or retain more of its elasticity, due to improved performance of skin cells. In some cases where skin becomes loose, due to rapid weight loss and/or aging, there have been some improvements in reversing and improving this as well. Combining the efforts of a ketogenic diet and the benefits of autophagy will greatly increase the anti-aging effects both have on the body, both inside and out.

Chapter 8: Frequently Asked Questions, Tips, and Encouragement for Long-Term Success and Benefits of the Autophagy Diet

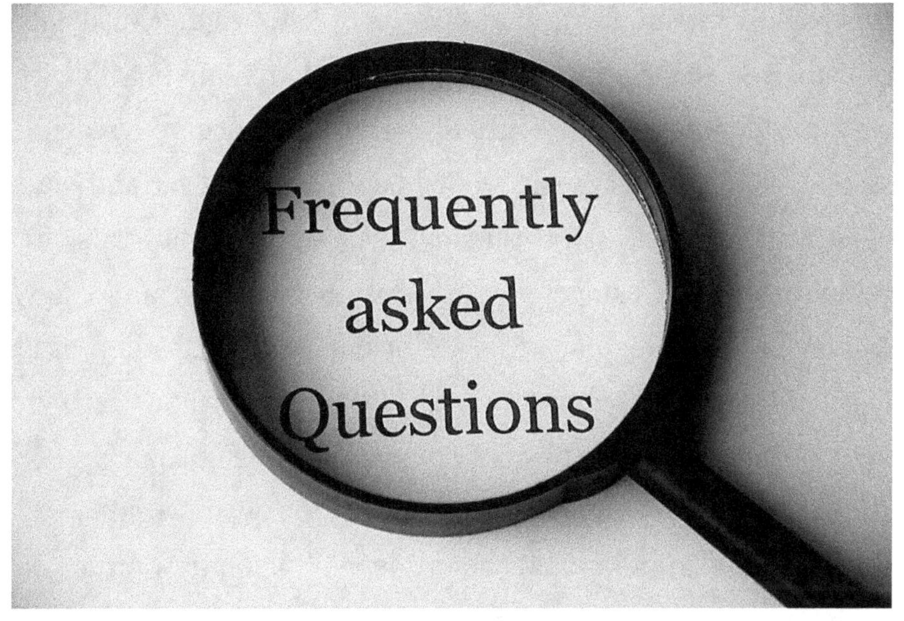

The autophagy diet or pathways to achieving a state of autophagy can be challenging and rewarding at the same time. In order to better understand and tackle some common issues and concerns associated with the benefits and struggles of shifting into a low carb diet and intermittent fasting, to produce results, the following frequently asked questions may prove helpful:

Q: How do I know when I reach autophagy?

A: The only way to detect the onset of autophagy is to verify the body's production of autophagosomes. While this is done in a lab for research purposes, it's not detectable through a home test kit. There are ways to detect if you are close to achieving this goal by testing for the production of ketones during a state of ketosis. Test strip kits can be purchased at many pharmacies over the counter and are usually accurate. Once you reach a state of ketosis, this means your body is burning fat and your cells will soon, if not already, search for materials for rebuilding. At this stage, you are close to reaching autophagy. Implementing a regular schedule of intermittent fasting, of at least 18 hours or more, in combination with low carb or ketogenic eating, is the best way to reach autophagy quickly.

Q: How often do I need to fast for autophagy to work?

A: This is an individual choice, depending on how often you wish to reach a state of autophagy, and will determine how often you fast. For example, fasting twice a week for 24-hours will help you reach this goal at least twice within the week. Longer fasts will take you to this goal as well and prolong the effects until you begin to eat again. Autophagy is not a process that occurs quickly, though once it is achieved, the benefits begin immediately. How often you choose to strive for this state is based on personal goals. Once or twice a week is a good start to see the results within a month.

Q: What is the best time frame for fasting to reach autophagy?

A: A 24-hour fast is an ideal goal for reaching the standard beginning of autophagy. Shorter fasting windows are a means to prepare and work towards this goal. If you choose to try dry fasting, your autophagy goal could be reached a bit sooner, between 18-24 hours, though using the 24-hour mark as a goal is based primarily on the findings that support a major increase in the production of autophagosomes at this stage. Expanding the fasting window to beyond the 24-hour window will continue the benefits of autophagy, once it is reached, though the benefits begin to plateau or lessen over time. In general, the 24-hour goal is the best option.

Q: What foods should I avoid within the eating window during intermittent fasting?

A: Low carb and ketogenic foods are strongly recommended, as they support the benefits of ketosis and autophagy, so eating anything outside of these options should be avoided unless you choose to add carbohydrates for energy at certain intervals. In general, avoid all refined and processed foods. This includes eliminating trans fats and chemically flavored foods that provide no nutritional benefit. While the occasional high carb treat isn't going to ruin a dietary plan, it can be habit-forming and addictive, especially if old eating habits included a lot of processed foods. Becoming accustomed to whole natural foods makes decisions a lot easier during eating windows.

Q: Can I exercise during a fast?

A: Yes. Exercise is good during a fast, as it speeds up towards autophagy, though if you feel faint or otherwise not comfortable engaging in high impact exercise, slow down. Yoga, stretching, and walking are all suitable ways to improve your fitness level while supporting your body's processes during a fast.

Tips for Achieving Autophagy Success

As long as you persevere and continue to improve, and work through the challenges of both ketogenic eating and intermittent fasting, there is no failure, only success. If you experience a setback, remember that it is a learning process. Making significant changes to the way you eat and live is not a simple procedure that can happen in one day. It is a lifestyle adjustment that can take weeks, months, and longer to fully implement, though the advantages are enormous and will sustain your health in the long-term. Keep in mind the following tips for achieving your goal towards autophagy:

- Document your progress and keep a list of foods that

work and don't fit within your plan. This will keep your grocery shopping easy.

- Give yourself time. If you break your fast early during the first, second, or more times, it's completely acceptable. Our bodies are good at adapting, but it takes longer for some of us than others.

- Allow yourself a break once in a while. Intermittent fasting doesn't have to be constant or even consistent if it doesn't always fit into your goals. You can take a break for days or a week at a time to enjoy a vacation or time away and jump into it at a later date.

Once you become used to the routine of low carb meals and intermittent fasting, taking a break now and again, as well as increasing your efforts will become easier and more enjoyable, especially once you begin to see the results of your effort. Achieving autophagy is a life-long process that can lead to a longer, healthier life for many people, and also build confidence and strength in your mind and body for a better quality of life.